Ismail Jatoi

Manfred Kaufmann

Jean Y. Petit

Atlas of Breast Surgery

Illustrator

Hans J. Schütze

Ismail Jatoi
Manfred Kaufmann
Jean Y. Petit

Atlas of Breast Surgery

With 132 Figures

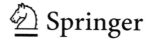

Springer

Ismail Jatoi M.D., Ph.D., F.A.C.S.
Uniformed Services
University of the Health Sciences
4301 Jones Bridge Road
Bethesda, Maryland 20814
USA

Professor Manfred Kaufmann M.D.
Klinik für Geburtshilfe und Gynäkologie
J. W. Goethe-Universität
Theodor-Stern-Kai 7
60590 Frankfurt
Germany

Jean Y. Petit M.D.
Istituto Europeo Di Oncologia
Via Ripamonti 435
20141 Milan
Italy

Library of Congress Control Number: 2005924216

ISBN-10 3-540-24351-8 Springer Berlin Heidelberg New York
ISBN-13 978-3-540-24351-9 Springer Berlin Heidelberg New York

Springer is a part of Springer Science+Business Media
springeronline.com
© Springer-Verlag Berlin Heidelberg 2006
Printed in Germany

Editor: Gabriele Schröder, Heidelberg, Germany
Desk Editor: Stephanie Benko, Heidelberg, Germany
Production: ProEdit GmbH, 69126 Heidelberg, Germany
Cover: Frido Steinen-Broo, EStudio, Calamar, Spain
Typesetting: K. Detzner, 67346 Speyer, Germany

Printed on acid-free paper   24/3151ML   5 4 3 2 1 0

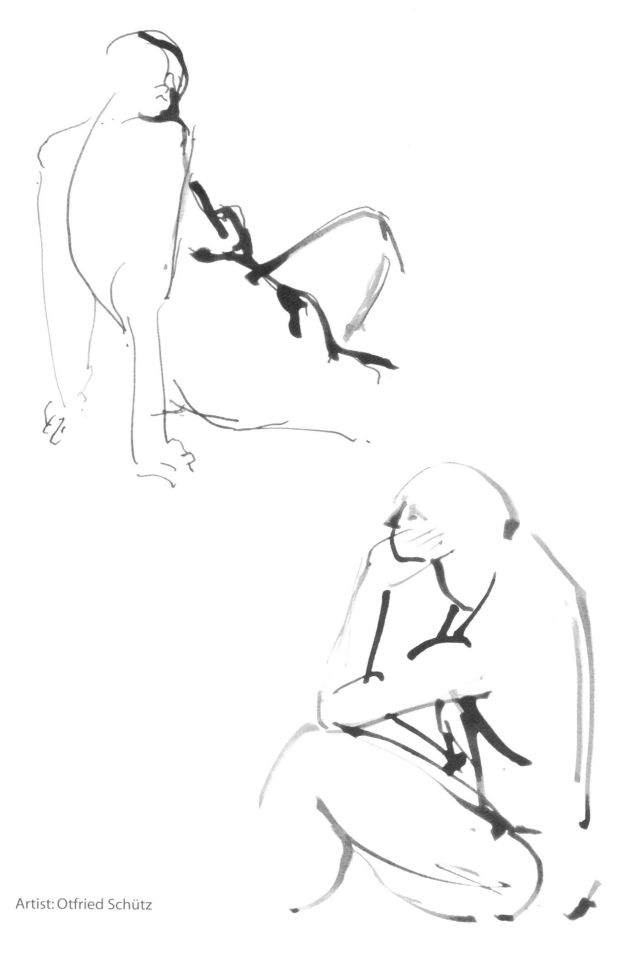

Artist: Otfried Schütz

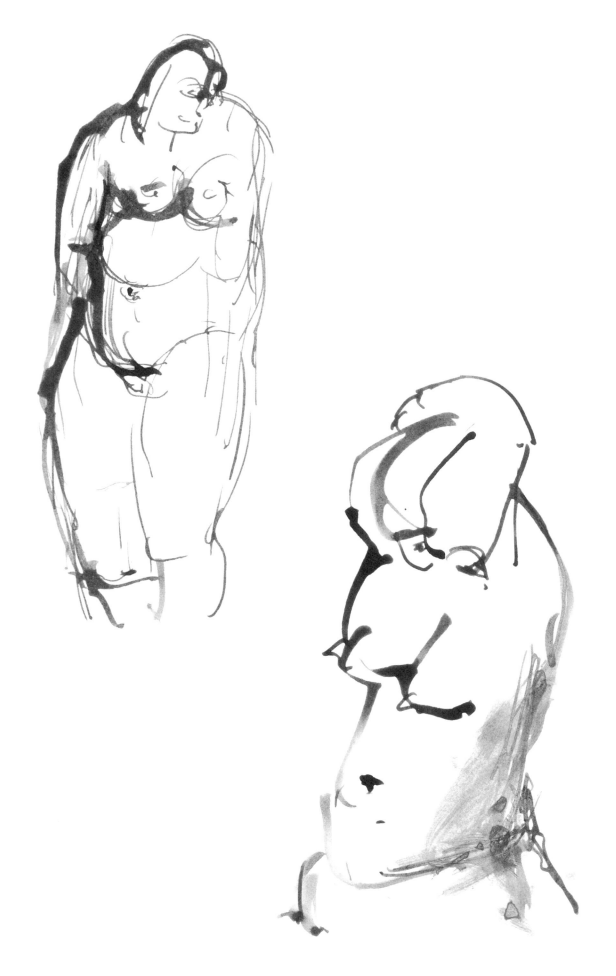

Preface

In recent years, there have been several important developments in the surgical management of breast diseases. We have witnessed the emergence of new techniques for tumor resection, reconstructive surgery, lymph node assessment, and cosmetic surgery, to name a few. Lately, the management of breast diseases has received considerable attention in the lay media, and patients today are not only demanding effective surgical treatments, but good cosmetic results as well. Thus, perhaps more than any other field, breast surgery has evolved into both a surgical science and an art. This atlas describes various surgical techniques for treating diseases of the breast, incorporating both the science and the art of this unique field.

This atlas provides a transatlantic perspective. The authors are from the United States, Germany, and Italy, and have a special interest in the treatment of breast diseases. Surgical techniques from both sides of the Atlantic are described, and this should appeal to readers who want to broaden their surgical repertoire. The management of both malignant and benign diseases of the breast is outlined, with illustrations to highlight key aspects of surgical techniques. Particular emphasis is placed on techniques that provide good cosmetic outcomes.

The completion of this atlas has required the collaborative effort of many individuals. We are particularly indebted to the editorial staff of the Springer-Verlag publishing company for their expert assistance and guidance. We wish to especially thank Ms. Stephanie Benko and Ms. Gabriele Schroeder of the Springer-Verlag office in Heidelberg, Germany, for their support in this endeavor and also Mrs. Sarah Price for the copy-editing. For the excellent illustrations and good cooperation we thank the artist Hans Jörg Schütze, Cologne, Germany. We sincerely hope that surgeons and surgically experienced gynecologists will find this atlas a valuable aid in the management of diseases of the breast.

Contents

Contents

Chapter 7
Plastic and Reconstructive Breast Surgery

Chapter 1

Historical Overview of Breast Surgery

The earliest reference to the surgical treatment of breast cancer can perhaps be found in what is now known as the "Edwin Smith Surgical Papyrus," a series of medical case presentations written in Egypt between 3000 and 2500 B.C. [1]. In those writings, it is clearly documented that physicians in ancient Egypt extirpated tumors of the breast. However, there was considerable controversy surrounding the surgical treatment of breast cancer throughout ancient times. Indeed, Hippocrates argued that breast cancer was a systemic disease, and that extirpation of the primary tumor made matters worse [2]. In about 400 B.C. he warned, "it is better not to excise hidden cancer, for those who are excised quickly perish; while they who are not excised live longer."

Similarly, Galen believed that breast cancer was a systemic disease, and promulgated the "humoral theory" to account for its pathogenesis [3]. Galen proposed that the breast tumor was a coagulum of black bile. He postulated that a woman's monthly menstrual flow relieved her of excess black bile, and that this accounted for the increased incidence of breast cancer among postmenopausal women. Yet, Galen strongly advocated surgery for the treatment of breast cancer. He urged surgeons to "excise a pathologic tumor in a circle in the region where it borders on the healing tissue." However, Galen's disciples often resorted to nonsurgical treatments, including special diets, purgation, venesection, and leaching. All were considered effective in getting rid of excess bile, and therefore acceptable options for the treatment of breast cancer.

In the eighteenth and nineteenth centuries, several surgeons promulgated a more aggressive surgical approach to the treatment of breast cancer (Fig. 1.1). Jean Louis Petit (1674–1750), Director of the French Surgical Academy, is credited with developing the first unified concept for the surgical treatment of breast cancer [4]. In his writings, published 24 years after his death, Petit suggests that "…the roots of cancer were the enlarged lymphatic glands; that the glands should be looked for and removed and that the pectoral fascia and even some fibers of the muscle itself should be dissected away rather than leave any doubtful tissue. The mammary gland too should not be cut into during the operation."

About the same time, the French surgeon LeDran challenged Galen's humoral theory. In 1757, he proposed that breast cancer was a local lesion that spread through the lymphatics [5]. Thus, LeDran argued that lymph node dissections should become an integral part of the surgical management of breast cancer. However, his views were not readily accepted. Indeed, Galen's humoral theory remained extremely popular throughout the eighteenth century, and many physicians were reluctant to discard it entirely,

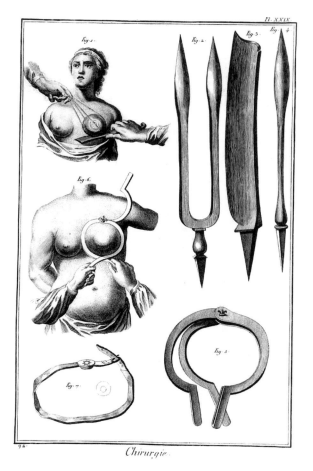

Fig. 1.1. Early instruments used for the removal of the breast and its tumors, as illustrated by Louis-Jacques Goussier, 1722–1792

preferring instead to simply modify it. For example, the English surgeon John Hunter proposed that breast cancer made its appearance where lymph coagulated, a hypothesis with obvious parallels to Galen's black bile theory [6]. Thus, Hunter and his disciples advocated the removal of enlarged lymph nodes in patients with primary breast cancer.

The modern surgical treatment of breast cancer has its origins in the mid nineteenth century. During this period, the German pathologist Rudolf Virchow (Fig. 1.2) studied the morbid anatomy of breast cancer [7]. He undertook careful postmortem dissections, and postulated that breast cancer arose from epithelial cells and then spread along fascial planes and lymphatic channels. These studies laid the scientific foundation for the surgical treatment of breast cancer from the late nineteenth to the later part of the twentieth century. In contrast to Galen, Virchow did not regard breast cancer as systemic at onset, but rather a local disease, amenable to cure with surgery.

Virchow's theory had a profound influence on the American surgeon William Halsted, who traveled through Europe in the late nineteenth century and studied with many of Virchow's pupils (Fig. 1.3). If we regard Virchow as the architect of the new cellular theory on breast cancer pathogenesis, then Halsted should be viewed as its engineer (Fig. 1.4). Shortly after returning to the United States, Halsted was appointed to the surgical faculty of the Johns Hopkins Hospital, where he described the radical mastectomy for the treatment of breast cancer [9]. This operation incorporated the tenets of Virchow's hypothesis. Thus, the tumor-containing breast, underlying pectoral muscles, and ipsilateral axillary contents were removed en bloc. In this manner, the lymphatic channels connecting the breast and axillary contents were extirpated, a clear acceptance of the teachings of Virchow, who had argued that cancer spreads along fascial planes and lymphatic channels, and a repudiation of the systemic hypothesis concerning breast cancer pathogenesis.

By the late nineteenth century, many surgeons throughout the United States and Europe had accept-

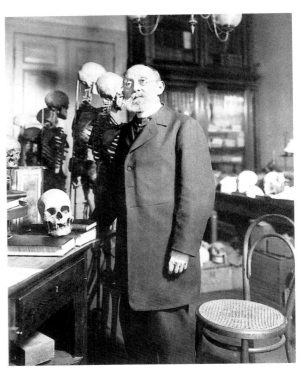

Fig. 1.2. The German pathologist Rudolph Virchow (1821–1902)

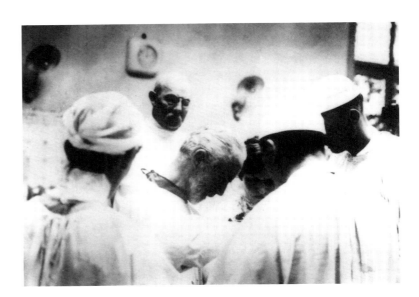

Fig. 1.3. In this photograph, the American surgeon William Halsted (*center*) is seen with his colleagues in Berlin

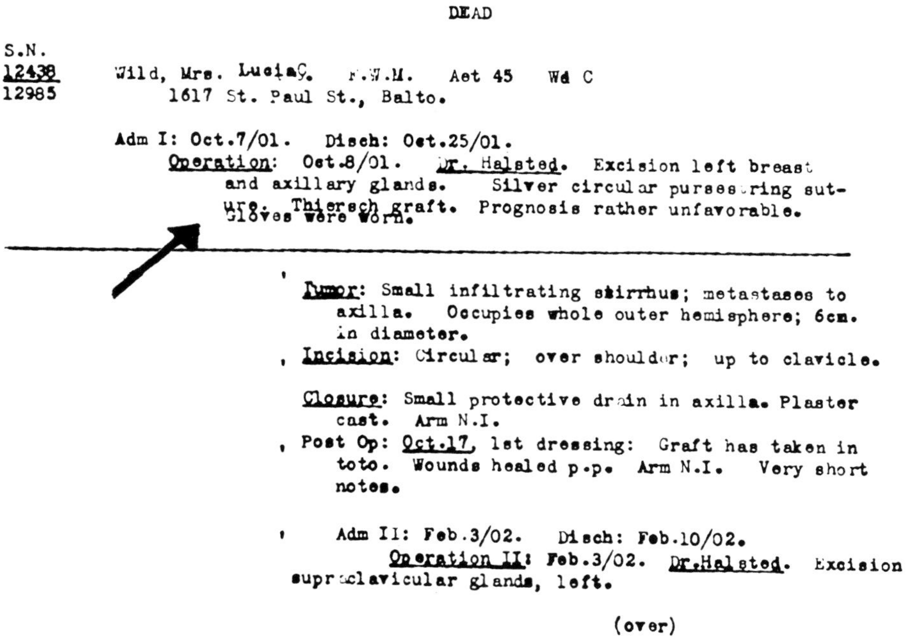

DEAD

```
S.N.
12438      Wild, Mrs. Lucia C.   r.W.M.   Aet 45   Wd C
12985         1617 St. Paul St., Balto.

        Adm I: Oct.7/01.   Disch: Oct.25/01.
           Operation:  Oct.8/01.  Dr. Halsted.  Excision left breast
              and axillary glands.   Silver circular pursee.ring sut-
              ure. Thiersch graft.  Prognosis rather unfavorable.
              Gloves were worn.
```

Fig. 1.4. Patient record by Dr. Halsted in 1901 with excellent documentation of staging and surgical procedure. Rubber gloves were used (from Lewinson [8])

```
              Tumor: Small infiltrating scirrhus; metastases to
                 axilla.  Occupies whole outer hemisphere; 6cm.
                 in diameter.
              Incision: Circular; over shoulder; up to clavicle.

              Closure: Small protective drain in axilla. Plaster
                 cast.  Arm N.I.
              Post Op: Oct.17, 1st dressing:  Graft has taken in
                 toto.  Wounds healed p.p.  Arm N.I.  Very short
                 notes.

              Adm II: Feb.3/02.   Disch: Feb.10/02.
                 Operation II: Feb.3/02.  Dr. Halsted.  Excision
              supraclavicular glands, left.

                            (over)
```

ed the Virchow/Halsted paradigm, and the operation that incorporated its tenets. The radical mastectomy was very effective in achieving local control of this disease, which, no doubt, contributed to its immense popularity. The transition from Galen's "systemic" paradigm to the Virchow/Halsted "local" paradigm was perhaps best summed up by Keen in a statement to the Cleveland Medical Society in 1894: "There is no question at all in the present day that [breast cancer] is of local origin. In my earlier professional life, it was one of the disputed points constantly coming up in medical society as to whether it was local or from the first a constitutional disease, and whether the latter it was said that no good could come from operating on the breast. But this question of local origin is no longer confronting us. It is a settled thing, a point won, and women must be taught that this brings hope to them" [10].

In 1948, Patey and Dyson of the Middlesex Hospital in London published a brief report describing a modification of the Halsted mastectomy [11]. In this "modified radical mastectomy," the pectoralis major muscle was preserved. The operation was less disfiguring, and the authors reported that its results were as good as those of the standard radical procedure. Many surgeons in the United States and Europe soon adopted this procedure as an alternative to the more radical Halsted operation. Indeed, a modified radical mastectomy (with preservation of both the pectoralis major and minor muscles) is still widely used today in the treatment of early breast cancer.

After World War II, McWhirter in Edinburgh advocated simple mastectomy and high-voltage x-ray therapy in the treatment of primary breast cancer. In 1948, he published his classic paper entitled "The value of simple mastectomy and radiotherapy in the treatment of cancer of the breast" in the *British Journal of Radiology* [12]. Although others had also suggested that radiotherapy be used in conjunction with surgery in the treatment of breast cancer, McWhirter was perhaps the most articulate spokesman for this treatment modality. He laid the foundations for the eventual use of radiotherapy in breast-conserving surgery. During the Halsted era, surgeons generally assumed that the radical mastectomy reduced breast cancer mortality. This assumption was based on the observation that the radical mastectomy was very effective in achieving local control of the disease, and it was believed that local control influenced survival. By the latter half of the twentieth century, some investigators were questioning this assumption. In 1962, Bloom et al. reported on the outcome of 250 patients with primary breast cancer who received absolutely no treatment [13]. These patients were diagnosed clinically between the years 1805 and 1933 at the Middlesex Hospital in London, and tissue diagnosis was established at autopsy. Henderson and Canellos compared the survival rate of these untreated patients from the Middlesex Hospital to those treated by radical mastectomy at the Johns Hopkins Hospital between the years 1889 and 1933 [14]. The survival curves of the two groups of patients were almost identical, suggesting that surgery contributed little to reducing breast cancer mortality. However, it is important to note that women in the late nineteenth and early twentieth centuries generally presented with locally advanced cancers, and many had distant metastasis at the time of presentation. In such patients, one would not expect local therapy (surgery) to have much impact on mortality. Yet, this might not necessarily hold true for women diagnosed with breast cancer today, who present earlier, without evidence of distant disease.

In recent years, several large randomized prospective trials have tested the tenets of the Halsted paradigm. Two trials, the National Surgical Adjuvant Breast Project-04 (NSABP-04) and the King's/Cambridge trials, randomized patients with clinically node-negative axilla to either early or delayed treatment of the axilla [15, 16]. The NSABP-04 trial was organized by Dr. Bernard Fisher of the National Surgical Breast and Bowel Project in Pittsburgh, USA, and the King's/Cambridge trial was organized by the Cancer Research Campaign (CRC) in the United Kingdom. In these trials, axillary treatment consisted of either surgical lymph node clearance or radiotherapy and was performed either at the time of mastectomy or delayed until tumor recurrence in the axilla. Both trials showed that the delayed treatment of the axilla does not adversely affect survival. Thus, contrary to Halsted's hypothesis, the axillary lymph nodes do not seem to serve as a nidus for the spread of cancer (Table 1.1).

Halsted had also postulated that breast cancer is a locally progressive disease, and that metastases occur by centrifugal and contiguous spread of the primary tumor in the breast. If this is indeed the case, then the extent of the mastectomy should influence survival. Over the last 30 years, this hypothesis has been tested in six randomized prospective trials [18–23]. These trials randomized patients with primary breast cancer to either a breast-conserving procedure (variously referred to as a lumpectomy, tylectomy, wide local excision, or quadrantectomy), or total mastectomy. The first of these six trials was conducted under the direction of Dr. Umberto Veronesi (Fig. 1.5) [21] at the Tumor Institute of Milan in Italy, and the largest trial (NSABP-06) was conducted by Dr. Bernard Fisher (Fig. 1.6) of the National Surgical Breast and Bowel Project in Pittsburgh, USA [22]. These trials showed that the risk of local recurrence increases following breast-conserving procedures, but the extent of the

Table 1.1. Comparison of Halstedian and Fisher hypotheses of tumor biology. The Fisher theory now is basis for all our treatment concepts, where adjuvant (postoperative) or neoadjuvant (preoperative) systemic treatment is standard of care (from Fisher [17])

Halstedian hypothesis	Fisher hypothesis
Tumors spread quickly in an orderly defined manner based upon mechanical considerations	There is no orderly pattern of tumor cell dissemination
Tumor cells traverse lymphatics to lymph nodes by direct extension supporting en bloc dissection	Tumor cells traverse lymphatics by embolization challenging the merit of en bloc dissection
The positive lymph node is an indicator of tumor spread and is the instigator of disease	The positive lymph node is an indicator of a host–tumor relationship which permits development of metastases rather than the instigator of distant disease
RLNs are barriers to the passage of tumor cells	RLNs are ineffective as barriers to tumor cell spread
RLNs are of anatomical importance	RLNs are of biological importance
The blood stream is of little significance as a route of tumor dissemination	The blood stream is of considerable importance in tumor dissemination
A tumor is autonomous of its host	Complex tumor–host interrelationships affect every facet of the disease
Operable breast cancer is a local–regional disease	Operable breast cancer is a systemic disease
The extent and nuances of operation are the dominant factors influencing patient outcome	Variations in local–regional therapy are unlikely to substantially affect survival

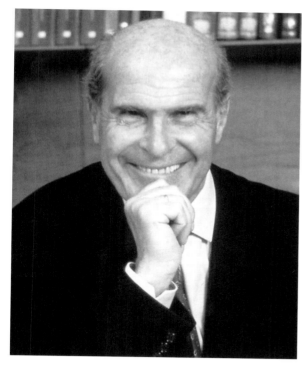

Fig. 1.5. Professor Umberto Veronesi of Milan, Italy

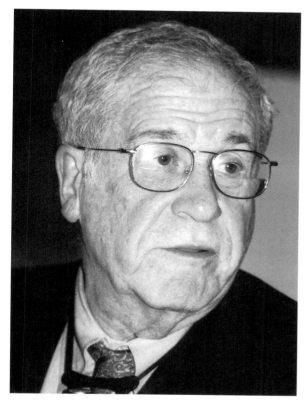

Fig. 1.6. Professor Bernard Fisher of Pittsburgh, USA

mastectomy does not influence survival, results that were inconsistent with the Halsted hypothesis.

The overall results of these randomized trials suggest that permutations in the surgical treatment of breast cancer have no impact on mortality. Ironically, these trials have led many investigators to once again conclude that breast cancer is a systemic disease at the time of diagnosis, a belief held by Galen and his disciples. Thus, over the last 2500 years, we seem to have come full circle in our thinking about the natural history of breast cancer!

Recently, there has been an increased emphasis on improving quality of life for those afflicted with breast cancer. Surgeons have played a very important role in this endeavor. The surgeon is often the first to discuss the diagnosis and treatment options with the patient, and effective communication skills can do much to allay anxiety and fear. Also, there is now a wider acceptance of breast reconstructive surgery as an important component in the overall management of breast cancer. Breast reconstruction can reduce the psychological trauma associated with mastectomy, particularly the sense of mutilation, depression, and misgivings concerning femininity. Surgeons throughout the world have described a wide array of reconstructive techniques, including the use of expanders, implants and tissue flaps [24]. In recent years, several prominent plastic surgeons in North American and Europe have taken a special interest in breast reconstructive surgery, and made it an integral part of plastic surgery training programs. Dr. John Bostwick of Emory University in Atlanta (Fig. 1.7) deserves much credit for developing the field in the United States.

Also, the sentinel lymph node biopsy technique has been studied as a means improving quality of life in patients with primary breast cancer [25]. The purpose of the sentinel lymph node biopsy is to stage patients with primary breast cancer, avoiding the morbidity of the traditional axillary lymph node dissection. Large trials are currently underway comparing the efficacy of sentinel node biopsy to the standard axillary lymph node dissection.

For centuries, the management of breast cancer was predicated on anecdotal experience and the results of retrospective studies. Today, it is largely based on the results of randomized, prospective clinical trials. These trials have shown that screening, adjuvant systemic therapy, and adjuvant radiotherapy can reduce breast cancer mortality. Surgeons have played a pivotal role in the design of many of these trials, and will undoubtedly continue to influence the design of future trials. The results of these clinical trials have clearly had a very favorable effect in improving the outcome for women with breast cancer.

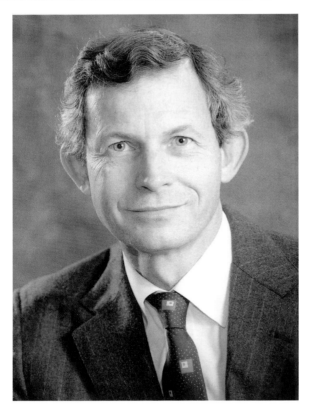

Fig. 1.7. Professor John Bostwick of Atlanta, USA

Indeed, since the early 1990s, breast cancer mortality rates have declined in many industrialized countries. Prior to this period, breast cancer mortality rates in these countries had either been stable or increasing for several decades. Thus, we are indeed making progress in the treatment of breast cancer [26, 27], and future progress will depend on the thoughtful planning of new clinical trials and patient participation in those trials.

References

1. Breasted JH (1930) The Edwin Smith surgical papyrus. The University of Chicago Press, Chicago, Ill.
2. Wood WC (1994) Progress from clinical trials on breast cancer. Cancer 74:2606–2609
3. Ariel IM (1987) Breast cancer, a historical review: is the past prologue? In: Ariel IM, Cleary JB (eds) Breast cancer diagnosis and treatment. McGraw-Hill, New York, pp 3–26
4. Robbins GF (1984) Clio chirurgica: the breast. Silvergirl, Austin, Tex.
5. LeDran HF (1757) Memoires avec un précis de plusieurs observations sur le cancer. Mem Acad R Chir 3:1–54
6. Martensen RL (1994) Cancer: medical history and the framing of a disease. J Am Med Assoc 271:1901
7. Virchow R (1863) Cellular pathology. Lippincott, Philadelphia, Pa.
8. Lewinson EF (1980) Changing concepts in breast cancer. Cancer 46:859–864
9. Halsted WS (1894) The results of operations for the cure of cancer of the breast performed at the Johns Hopkins Hospital from June 1889 to January 1894. Ann Surg 20:497–455
10. Keen WW (1894) Amputation of the female breast. Cleve Med Gaz 10:39–54
11. Patey DH, Dyson WH (1948) The prognosis of carcinoma of the breast in relation to the type of operation performed. Br J Cancer 2:7
12. McWhirter R (1948) The value of simple mastectomy and radiotherapy in the treatment of cancer of the breast. Br J Radiol 21:599
13. Bloom HJG, Richardson WW, Harries EJ (1962) Natural history of untreated breast cancer (1805–1933). Br Med J 2:213–221
14. Henderson IC, Canellos EP (1980) Cancer of the breast: the past decade. N Engl J Med 302:17–30
15. Fisher B, Redmond C, Fisher ER et al (1985) Ten-year results of a randomized clinical trial comparing radical mastectomy and total mastectomy with or without radiation. N Engl J Med 312:674–681
16. Cancer Research Campaign Working Party (1980) Cancer Research Campaign (King's/Cambridge) trial for early breast cancer. Lancet ii:55–60
17. Fisher B (1981) A commentary on the role of the surgeon in primary breast cancer. Breast Cancer Res Treat 1:17–26
18. Blichert-Toft M, Rose C, Andersen JA, Overgaard M et al (1992) Danish randomized trial comparing breast conservation therapy with mastectomy: six years of life-table analysis. J Natl Cancer Inst Monogr 11:19–35
19. Arriagada R, Le MG, Rochard F et al (1996) Conservative treatment versus mastectomy in early breast cancer: patterns of failure with 15 years of follow-up data. J Clin Oncol 14:1558–1564
20. van Dongen JA, Voogd AC, Fentiman IS, Legrand C, Sylvester RJ et al (2000) Long-term results of a randomized trial comparing breast-conserving therapy with mastectomy: European organization for research and treatment of cancer 10801 trial. J Natl Cancer Inst 92:1143–1150
21. Veronesi U, Cascinelli N, Mariani L, Greco M, Saccozzi R, Luini A et al (2002) Twenty-year follow-up of a randomized study comparing breast-conserving surgery with radical mastectomy for early breast cancer. N Engl J Med 347:1227–1232
22. Fisher B, Anderson S, Bryant J, Margolese RG et al (2002) Twenty-year follow-up of a randomized trial comparing total mastectomy, lumpectomy, and lumpectomy plus irradiation for the treatment of invasive breast cancer. N Engl J Med 347:1233–1241
23. Poggi MM, Danforth DN, Sciuto LC, Smith SL, Steinberg SM et al (2003) Eighteen-year results in the treatment of early breast carcinoma with mastectomy versus breast conservation therapy. Cancer 98:697–702
24. Bostwick J (1990) Plastic and reconstructive breast surgery. Quality Medical, St. Louis, Mo.
25. Giuliano AE (1996) Sentinel lymphadenectomy in primary breast carcinoma: an alternative to routine axillary dissection. J Surg Oncol 62:75–77
26. Goldhirsch A, Wood WC, Gelber RD et al (2003) Meeting highlights: updated international expert consensus on the primary therapy of early breast cancer. J Clin Oncol 21:3357–3365
27. Kaufmann M, v. Minckwitz G, Smith R, Valero V, Gianni L et al (2003) International expert panel on the use of primary (preoperative) systemic treatment of operable breast cancer: review and recommendations. J Clin Oncol 21:2600–2608

Chapter 2

Anatomy

2.1 Surface Anatomy of the Breast

The breasts are modified skin glands, located on the anterior and also partly the lateral aspects of the thorax. Each breast extends superiorly to the second rib, inferiorly to the sixth costal cartilage, medially to the sternum, and laterally to the mid-axillary line (Fig. 2.1). The nipple–areola complex is located between the fourth and fifth ribs. Natural lines of skin tension, known as Langer lines, extend outwards circumferentially from the nipple–areola complex. The lines of Langer assume particular clinical significance for the surgeon, when determining where to place the incision for breast biopsies, as discussed later in this text.

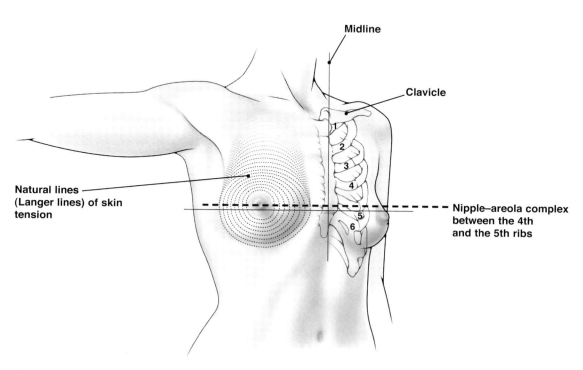

Fig. 2.1. Surface anatomy of the breast

2

2.2 Breast Development

The mammary gland is primarily derived from epidermal thickenings that develop along the ventral surface of the body, along the so-called milk line. In the female, most of the development of the breast occurs after birth. In contrast, in the male, no further breast development occurs after birth. In the female, growth and branching of the mammary glands progress slowly during the prepubertal years (Fig. 2.2a). Then, development of the mammary glands dramatically increases at puberty (Fig. 2.2b), with further branching of ducts, formation of acini buds, and a dramatic proliferation of interductal stroma. This results in the formation of a breast bud. The sudden appearance of a breast bud on the chest wall is sometimes a cause for concern. It is not uncommon for mothers to bring their daughters in for medical evaluation after finding a new lump on the chest wall. The surgeon should exercise great caution when considering biopsy of any mass on the chest wall in a young girl prior to the development of mature breasts. Excision of a breast bud will prevent development of a mammary gland.

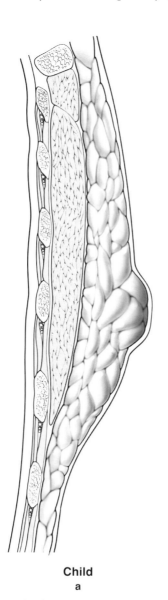

Child

a

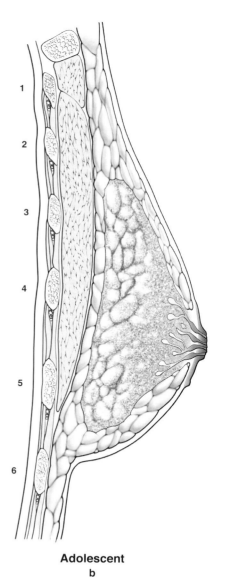

Adolescent

b

Fig. 2.2a–d. Breast development. a In a prepubertal girl, the mammary glands grow and branch slowly. b In adolescence the mammary glands develop rapidly, with the growth of the duct system influenced by estrogen and progesterone

As indicated previously, only the major breast ducts are formed at birth, and the mammary glands remain essentially undeveloped until puberty. At puberty, the mammary glands develop rapidly, primarily due to the proliferation of stromal and connective tissue around the ducts. Growth of the duct system occurs through the influence of estrogen and progesterone, secreted by the ovaries during puberty (Fig. 2.2c). Only at the time of pregnancy does the breast achieve complete structural maturation and full functional activity. During pregnancy, the intralobular ducts develop rapidly, forming buds that become alveoli, and the stromal/glandular proportions in the breast are reversed. By the end of pregnancy, the breast is composed almost entirely of glandular units separated by small amounts of stromal tissue. Following lactation, the acini atrophy, ductal structres shrink, and the whole breast markedly diminishes in size.

With the onset of menopause, the acini regress further, with loss of both interlobular and intralobular connective tissue. With time, the acini structures may be completely absent from the breast in the postmenopausal female. Thus, the morphologic appearance of the breast in postmenopausal women is much different from that of women during their premenopausal years. During the postmenopausal years, both the ductal structures and connective tissue of the breasts are markedly diminished in size (Fig. 2.2d).

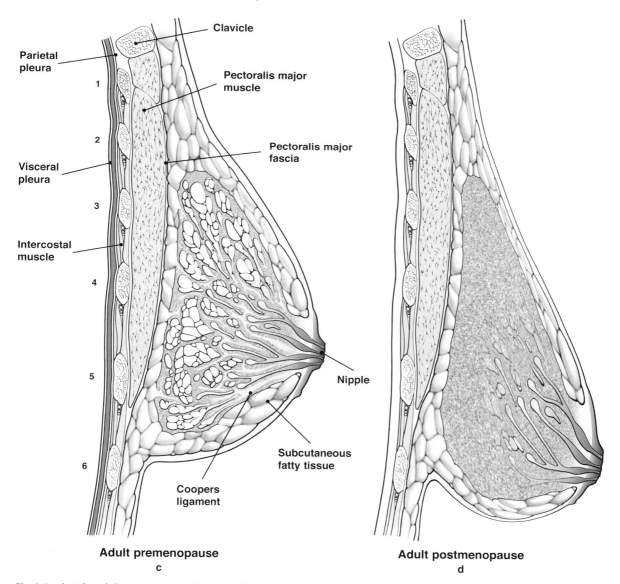

Adult premenopause
c

Adult postmenopause
d

Fig. 2.2c, d. c The adult premenopausal breast. d The adult postmenopausal breast. Ribs are numbered in b and c

2

2.3 Organization of the Ductal-Lobular System, and its Diseases

Figure 2.3 illustrates the ductal-lobular system of the breast, and the anatomical location of some common pathological lesions. The ductal system contains numerous lobules with acini. Each lobule feeds into a terminal duct, which, in turn, feeds into a segmental duct. The segmental ducts ultimately feed into collecting ducts, and about 15–20 of these converge under the areola on to the surface of the nipple through separate orifices.

The three most common causes of a discrete breast mass in a woman are cysts, fibroadenomas, and carcinomas. Cysts and fibroadenomas develop within lobules while carcinomas develop in the terminal ducts. Common causes of nipple discharge are papillomas and duct ectasia, and these develop in the segmental ducts. Nipple adenomas also develop in the segmental ducts, near their openings in the nipple. Paget's disease of the breast refers to excoriation of the skin in the nipple–areola complex. This generally indicates the presence of an underlying carcinoma of the breast. Half of these cases are attributable to ductal carcinoma in situ and the other half to invasive carcinoma.

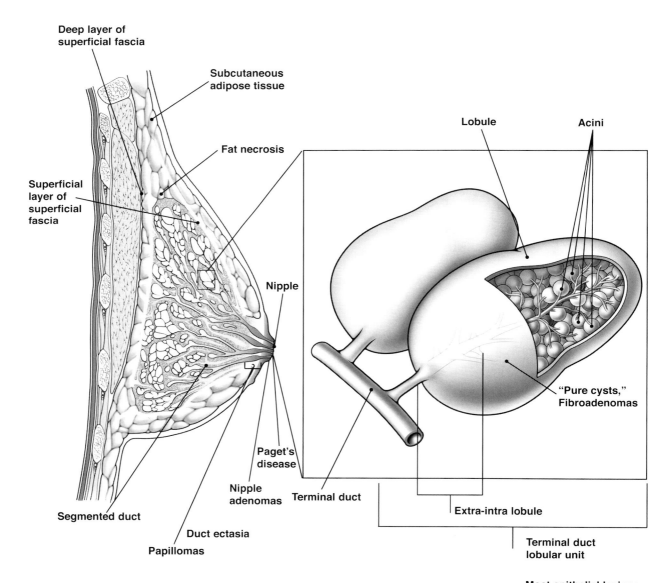

Fig. 2.3. Organization of the ductal-lobular system and its diseases

2.4 Blood Supply of the Breast

The blood supply of the breast is derived primarily from the internal mammary artery (internal thoracic artery), and the lateral thoracic artery (Fig. 2.4). Both these arteries originate from the axillary artery and then enter the breast from the superomedial and superolateral aspects, respectively. Branches of these arteries anastomose with one another. Additionally, the internal mammary artery gives rise to the posterior intercostal arteries, and branches of the intercostal arteries penetrate the deep surface of the breast.

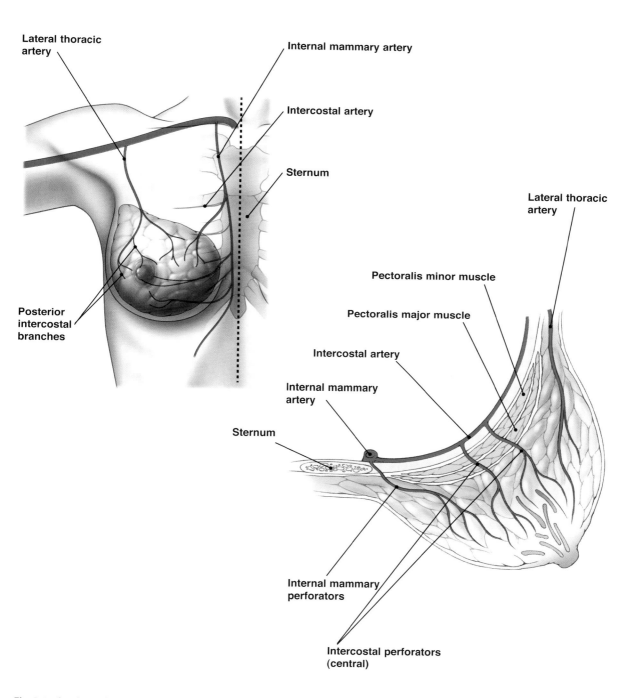

Fig. 2.4. Blood supply of the breast

2.5 Anatomy of the Axilla

The axilla is bound medially with the chest wall, laterally by the latissimus dorsi muscle, superiorly by the axillary vein, posteriorly by the subscapularis muscle, and inferiorly by the interdigitation of the latissimus dorsi and serratus anterior muscles (Fig. 2.5a, b). The axilla is divided into three levels, defined by their anatomical relationship to the pec-

toralis minor muscle. These axillary levels are of particular clinical significance when discussing the extent of axillary dissection for carcinoma of the breast. Axillary tissue that is lateral to the lateral border of the pectoralis minor muscle is defined as level I; posterior and between the lateral and medial borders of the muscle is level II; and medial to the medial border of the muscle is level III. The surgical relevance of these levels is discussed later, in Sect. 6.4.

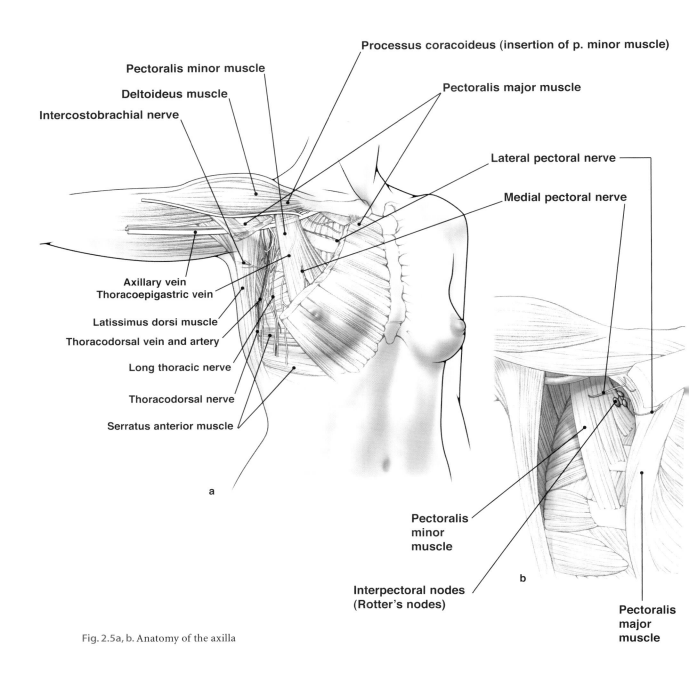

Fig. 2.5a, b. Anatomy of the axilla

There are several clinically important structures within the axilla. Between the pectoralis major and minor muscles are the interpectoral lymph nodes (Rotter's nodes). These nodes are usually found on the posterior surface of the pectoralis major muscle. The lateral pectoral nerve also courses along the posterior surface of the pectoralis major muscle, and injury to this nerve will result in atrophy of this muscle. The medial pectoral nerve, which has a Y shape, innervates the inferior–lateral aspect of the pectoralis major muscle and should be carefully preserved during dissection.

The second cutaneous intercostobrachial nerve lies approximately 1 cm inferior to the axillary vein, and runs in a medial–lateral direction. The long thoracic nerve, which innervates the serratus anterior muscle, can be identified just posterior to the intercostobrachial nerve at the second interspace. The long thoracic nerve follows the curve of the chest wall inferiorly and posteriorly, until it divides into branches that insert into the serratus anterior muscle at about the level of the fourth or fifth rib. Although the long thoracic nerve generally runs along the serratus anterior muscle, it may also lie more laterally in the axillary tissue. Therefore, the nerve should be identified before proceeding with axillary dissection immediately lateral to the serratus anterior muscle. It is also important to note that the long thoracic nerve runs in a superior–inferior direction, and is always posterior to the intercostal nerves (which run in a medial–lateral direction). Thus, any surgical dissection anterior to the intercostal nerves will safely preserve the long thoracic nerve. Transection of the long thoracic nerve results in a "winged scapula."

The thoracodorsal nerve innervates the latissimus dorsi muscle. Superiorly, it lies posterior to the lateral thoracic (thoracoepigastric) vein. It then takes an inferolateral course, lying on the subscapular muscle, accompanied by the subscapular vessels, and enters the medial aspect of the latissimus dorsi muscle. Thus, dissection along the lateral or anterior aspects of the latissimus dorsi muscle will avoid damage to the thoracodorsal nerve.

2.6 Latissimus Dorsi Muscle and Related Muscles

The latissimus dorsi muscle forms the lateral border of the axilla (Fig. 2.6). It is an important landmark in the surgical treatment of primary breast cancer, and is often used in breast reconstructive surgery following mastectomy for cancer (the latissimus dorsi flap). The relevance of the latissimus dorsi muscle is discussed later, in Sect. 7.6

The latissimus dorsi muscle originates from the thoracic vertebrae (T7–T12), the iliac crest and lumbar and sacral spines (by way of the thoracolumbar fascia), and the lower three or four ribs. The latissimus dorsi muscle inserts on the floor of the intertubercular groove. The muscle functions as a medial rotator, and also serves to adduct and extend the arm.

There are several muscles that lie in close relationship to the latissimus dorsi muscle. The deltoid is a thick, triangular muscle that arises from the lateral third of the clavicle, the acromion, and the lower edge of the scapular spine. It inserts on the deltoid tuberosity, which is located on the lateral aspect of the humeral midshaft. The deltoid facilitates the abduction, medial rotation, and lateral rotation of the arm. The teres major muscle originates from the inferior angle and the dorsal surface of the scapula. It inserts on the crest of the lesser tubercle of the humerus and facilitates adduction of the arm and serves as a medial rotator. Finally, the trapezius muscle is a flat, triangular muscle that extends over the back of the neck and upper thorax. It is attached to the medial third of the superior nuchal line, external occipital protuberance, and the spinous processes from C7 to T12. The trapezius works in conjunction with other muscles to steady the scapula.

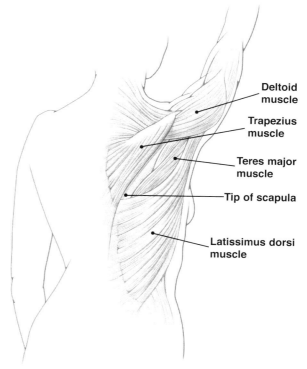

Deltoid muscle

Trapezius muscle

Teres major muscle

Tip of scapula

Latissimus dorsi muscle

Fig. 2.6. Latissimus dorsi muscle and related muscles

2

2.7 Anterior View of Latissimus Dorsi Muscle and Blood Supply (Pectoralis Major Muscle Removed)

The surgeon should become familiar with the blood supply of the latissimus dorsi muscle because of its applications in breast reconstructive surgery (Fig. 2.7). The subscapular artery originates as a branch from the axillary artery, and soon branches to give off the circumflex scapular artery and the thoracodorsal artery. One or two veins and the thoracodorsal nerve join the thoracodorsal artery, forming a neurovascular pedicle. This pedicle enters the latissimus dorsi muscle on its medial surface, approximately 6–12 cm from the subscapular artery.

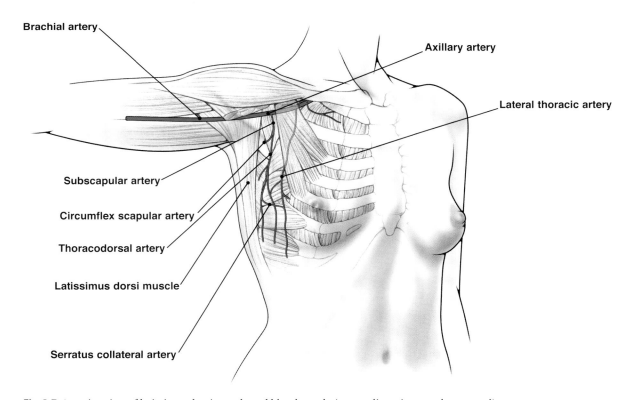

Fig. 2.7. Anterior view of latissimus dorsi muscle and blood supply (pectoralis major muscle removed)

2.8 Anterior Abdominal Wall and Blood Supply

The rectus abdominis muscle, like the latissimus dorsi muscle, is important in breast reconstructive sur-gery, as discussed later, in Sect. 7.6. Specifically, it is used in the creation of TRAM (transverse rectus ab-dominis muscle) flaps. The rectus abdominis muscle originates from the cartilage of the 5th, 6th, and 7th ribs and the xiphoid process. It inserts in front of the symphysis and body of the pubic bone (Fig. 2.8).

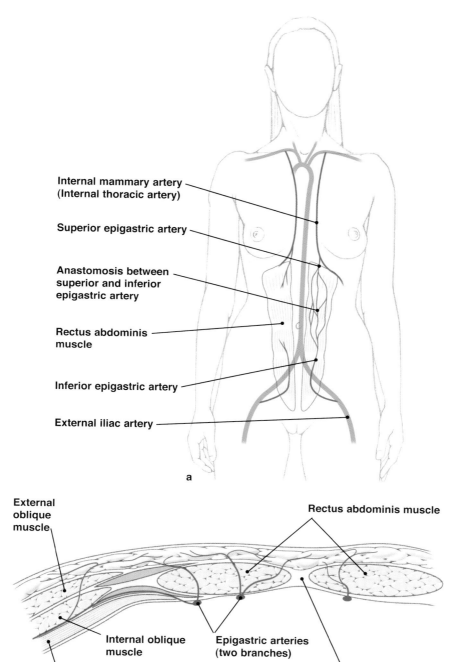

Internal mammary artery
(Internal thoracic artery)

Superior epigastric artery

Anastomosis between
superior and inferior
epigastric artery

Rectus abdominis
muscle

Inferior epigastric artery

External iliac artery

a

External
oblique
muscle

Rectus abdominis muscle

Internal oblique
muscle

Epigastric arteries
(two branches)

b   Transversus abdominis muscle

Linea alba

Fig. 2.8a, b. Anterior abdominal wall and blood supply

2

The external oblique muscle ends in an aponeurosis that runs anterior to the rectus abdominis muscle. The internal oblique muscle ends in an aponeurosis that splits into anterior and posterior layers. The anterior layer passes in front of the rectus abdominis muscle and fuses with the aponeurosis of the external oblique muscle. The posterior layer passes behind the rectus abdominis muscle above the arcuate line. Below the arcuate line, this layer also passes in front of the rectus abdominis muscle. Finally, above the arcuate line, the transversus abdominis muscle ends in an aponeurosis that runs behind the rectus abdominis muscle. Below the arcuate line, the aponeurosis of the transversus abdominis muscle passes in front of the rectus abdominis muscle. Thus, above the arcuate line, the posterior layer of the rectus sheath is formed by the aponeurosis of the transversus abdominis and internal oblique muscles. Below the arcuate line, the posterior layer of the rectus sheath is formed by the fascia transversalis.

Within the rectus sheath, the superior epigastric artery and the inferior epigastric artery form an anastomosis (Fig. 2.8b). The inferior epigastric artery enters the rectus sheath at the arcuate line. It should be noted that the superior epigastric artery is the terminal branch of the internal thoracic (internal mammary) artery, and the inferior epigastric artery is a branch of the external iliac artery.

Figure 2.9 shows the location of primary breast cancer and metastases.

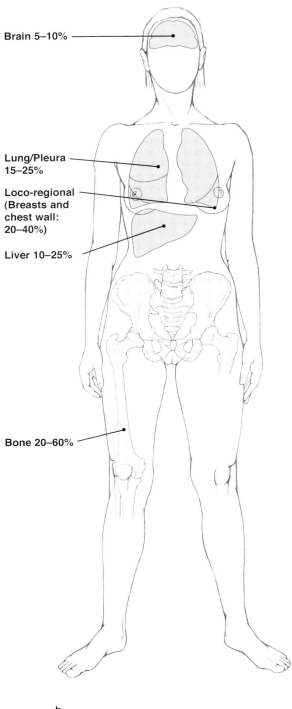

Brain 5–10%

Lung/Pleura 15–25%

Loco-regional (Breasts and chest wall: 20–40%)

Liver 10–25%

Bone 20–60%

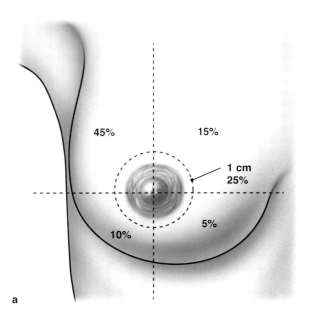

45%   15%

1 cm 25%

10%   5%

a   b

Fig. 2.9a–c. Location of primary breast cancer and their metastases. a Location of primary breast cancer. b Localization of first site of metastases

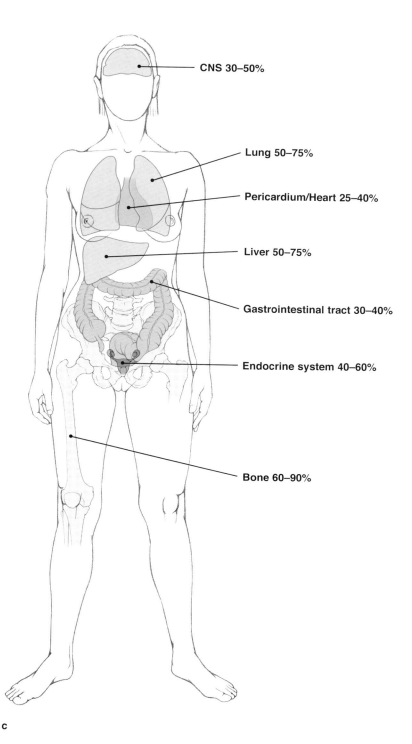

CNS 30–50%

Lung 50–75%

Pericardium/Heart 25–40%

Liver 50–75%

Gastrointestinal tract 30–40%

Endocrine system 40–60%

Bone 60–90%

c

Fig. 2.9c. Localization of recurrence at autopsy

Chapter 3

Diagnostic Procedures

3.1 Fine Needle Aspiration

Fine needle aspiration (FNA) is a quick way to diagnose malignancy in a patient with a breast mass. First, the skin is cleaned with rubbing alcohol. The surgeon then fixes the tumor with his or her hand, using either the thumb and index finger or index finger and middle finger. A syringe attached to a 21-gauge needle is then placed into the breast mass while suction on the syringe is maintained (Figs. 3.1, 3.2, 3.3). We generally use a 20-ml syringe for this purpose. The needle is passed through the breast mass in various directions (but never brought out of the mass), while maintaining suction on the syringe.

Suction is then released and the needle brought out of the breast mass. The tissue debris on the needle and tip of the syringe is sprayed onto glass slides, using the syringe plunger. The slides are air-dried and subsequently stained and processed by the pathologist (Fig. 3.5a, b) to assess for the presence of malignant cells. If malignant cells are identified, this usually indicates the presence of invasive carcinoma, because ductal carcinoma in situ (DCIS) is rarely palpable, and generally presents as an abnormality seen only on mammogram. Yet, to completely exclude the possibility of DCIS, an excisional biopsy is required.

When assessing a breast mass for malignancy, FNA has a very low false-positive rate. However, the false-negative rate is much higher. Therefore, if no malignant cells are detected on FNA (Fig. 3.5a), many surgeons will proceed with excisional biopsy to definitely exclude the possibility of cancer. However, in most cases FNA should be performed under ultrasound guidance (Fig. 3.4).

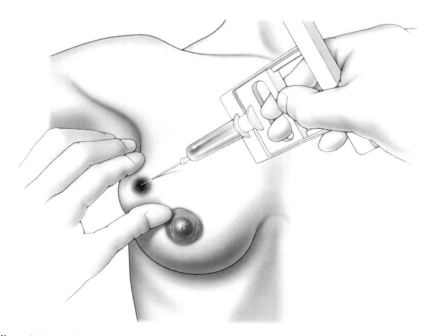

Fig. 3.1. Fine needle aspiration of a palpable breast mass

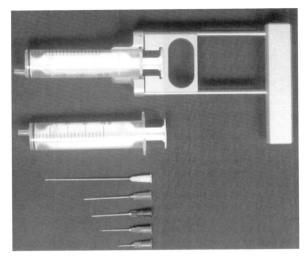

Equipment for punction of cysts:

Syringes 20 ml
Cameco syringe pistol (optionally)
Needle (20 g, 7 cm preferred)

Fig. 3.2. Equipment required for the punction of breast cysts

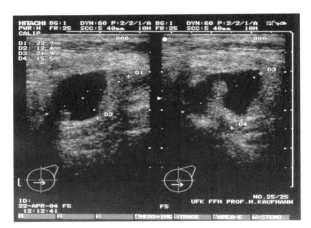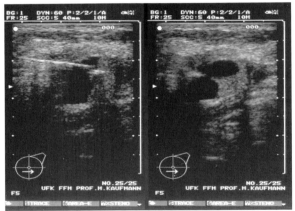

Fig. 3.3. FNA of a 63-year-old patient presenting with a new finding after TRAM flap surgery for invasive breast cancer

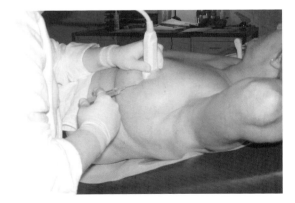

Fig. 3.4. Ultrasound guided biopsy after local anasthesia

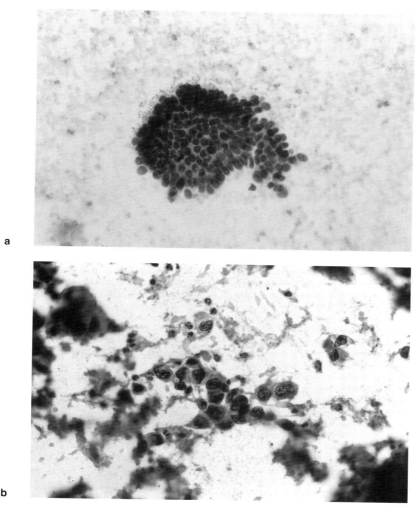

a

b

Fig. 3.5a, b. a Fine needle puncture: normal breast epithelial complex (× 400). b Fine needle puncture: tumor cells from solid breast cancer (× 400)

3

3.2 Core Needle Biopsy[1]

The technique of core needle biopsy can be applied to both palpable and nonpalpable breast lesions. If the lesion is palpable, image guidance is generally not necessary. The skin overlying the breast mass is cleaned with rubbing alcohol and local anesthetic is injected around the intended biopsy site A small cut is made on the skin overlying the breast mass using an 11-blade knife, and the tip of the biopsy instrument (Fig. 3.6) is placed against the mass. The breast mass is then stabilized with one hand, and the biopsy instrument fired with the other hand. Caution should be used when stabilizing the lesion by hand. The biopsy needle is thrust forward about 2 cm when fired, and can injure the assisting hand. The tissue samples are placed in formaldehyde, and submitted to pathology. The surgeon should inspect the tissue samples in the formaldehyde. If the tissue floats, this generally indicates that the sample is not adequate, and additional tissue should be obtained. After obtaining adequate tissue, a band-aid is placed over the cut.

For nonpalpable lesions, visualization with either ultrasound or mammography is required to obtain core biopsy samples (Fig. 3.7).

When performing an ultrasound-guided biopsy, local anesthetic is injected around the intended biopsy site. A small incision is made with a number 11-blade scalpel to allow entry of the biopsy needle into the breast. The entry point should be made about 1–2 cm away from the ultrasound transducer probe, which allows the surgeon to visualize the breast lesion. The surgeon should test-fire the biopsy gun and become familiar with its firing mechanism before placing the spring-loaded needle into the breast tissue.

The surgeon can generally hold the ultrasound probe with one hand and manipulate the spring-loaded needle with the other hand. However, it is of-ten helpful to have a technician stabilize the ultrasound probe, giving the surgeon additional flexibility to manipulate the biopsy instrument. The needle should be directed to the edge of the area of concern, and photo-documentation of the image completed. The patient should then be warned that the biopsy instrument is about to be fired. The instrument is then fired, obtaining the necessary core biopsy samples of the breast lesion. After completing the procedure, the biopsy specimens are placed in formaldehyde and sent to the pathologist, and a band-aid is placed over the breast wound.

A vacuum-assisted breast biopsy system and the result are shown in Fig. 3.8, 3.9, 3.10.

The term "stereotactic breast biopsy" refers to a method of sampling (Figs. 3.8, 3.9) breast lesions that are visualized mammographically (Fig. 3.10). The mammograms should be carefully reviewed to determine the best directional approach to the lesion. A computer calculates the coordinates for horizontal, vertical, and depth axes, so as to direct the attached core needle device to the targeted lesion on the breast (Fig. 3.11). The patient is positioned prone on the procedure table, with the breast in the dependent position through an aperture on the stereotactic table (Fig. 3.12, 3.13). The skin overlying the breast is cleaned with povidone-iodine (Betadine®) solution or alcohol, and the needle entry site should be infiltrated with local anesthetic prior to making a small skin incision with an 11-blade knife. The needle is then manually advanced to the appropriate depth as calibrated by a computer, and stereo images are taken to ensure correct position of the needle tip in relation to the breast lesion. The spring-loaded needle is then fired into the breast lesion, and the appropriate location of the core biopsy confirmed with repeated stereo images. The core biopsy samples obtained in this manner (Fig. 3.14) are submitted to pathology together with radiographs (Fig. 3.15, 3.16, 3.17) and a band-aid placed over the small cut on the breast.

---

[1] (Illustrations are courtesy of Christine Solbach MD, Department of Obstetrics and Gynecology, and Thomas Diebold MD, Department of Radiology, Goethe University, Frankfurt, Germany)

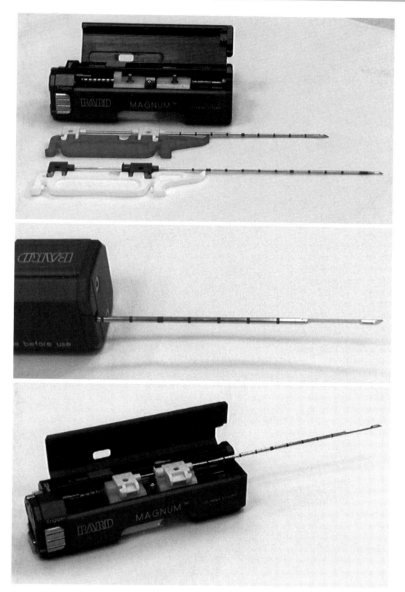

Fig. 3.6. High-speed core-cut biopsy instrument. The example shown is an Angiomed BARD MAGNUM, with 12/14 or 16 g probes, length 100 mm, biopsy diameter 1.9 mm

3

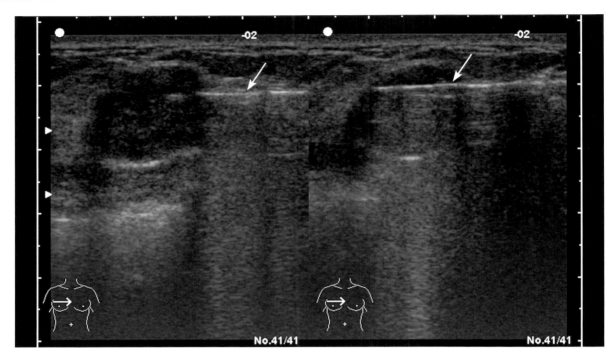

Fig. 3.7. When taking high-speed core-cut biopsy samples of nonpalpable and palpable breast masses, visualization with ultrasound may be required

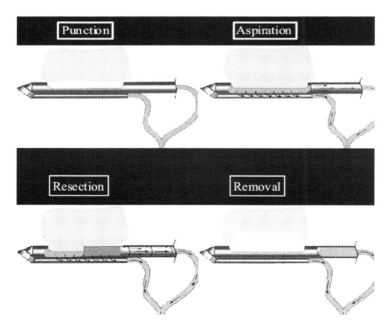

Fig. 3.8. The vacuum-assisted breast biopsy system allows punction, aspiration, resection, and removal of breast lesions that are visualized mammographically throughout the procedure (Ethicon Endo-Surgery)

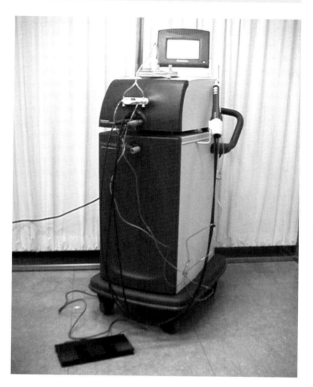
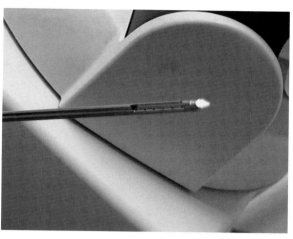

Fig. 3.9. A vacuum-assisted percutaneous biopsy device and biopsy needle (brand name Mammotome®, manufactured by Johnson and Johnson Ethicon Endo-Surgery)

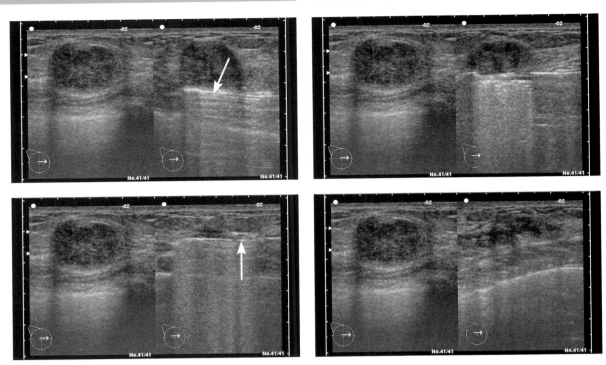

Fig. 3.10. Using the vacuum-assisted breast biopsy system, the probe is positioned at the lesion. It vacuums, cuts, and removes tissue samples, which are passed through the probe's hollow chamber into a collection tray. This allows for multiple samples to be collected while only one incision into the breast is made. At the end hematoma remains visable

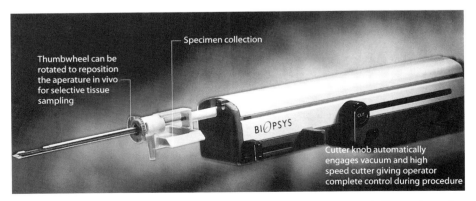

Fig. 3.11. The core needle device of the vacuum-assisted breast biopsy system, showing the hollow probe and specimen collection tray

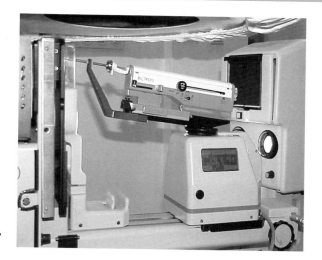

Fig. 3.12. The vacuum-assisted biopsy system shown in place, below the aperture in the stereotactic table

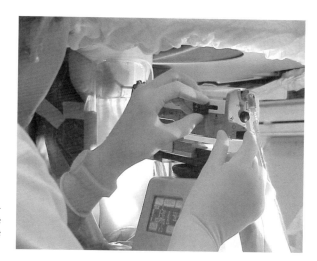

Fig. 3.13. The surgeon or radiologist can rotate the thumb-wheel of the vacuum-assisted biopsy probe, moving it to the correct position for the next biopsy sample, to allow multiple samples to be taken with just one breast incision

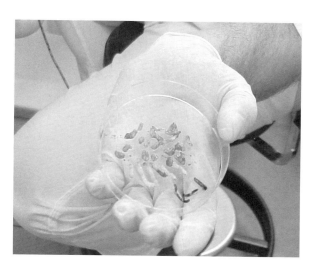

Fig. 3.14. Multiple core biopsy samples obtained following one vacuum-assisted biopsy procedure

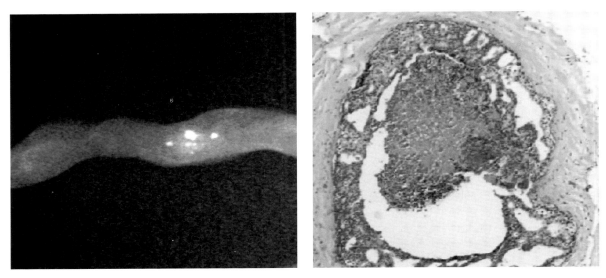

Fig. 3.15. Ductal carcinoma in situ (*DCIS*) in a specimen obtained by vacuum-assisted biopsy

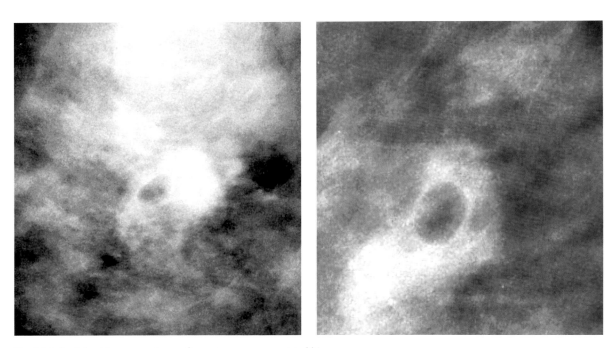

Fig. 3.16. Excision biopsy specimen after prior vacuum-assisted biopsy

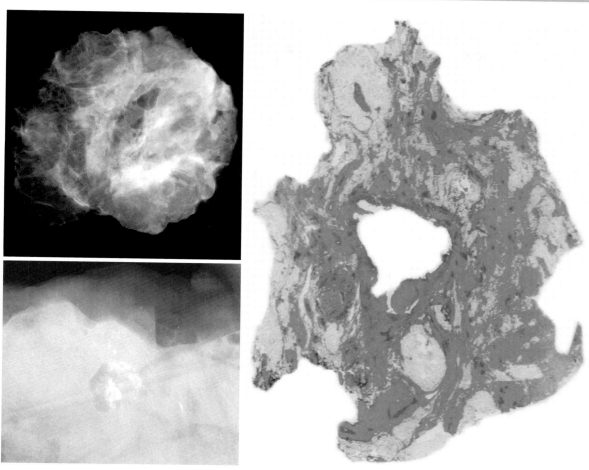

Fig. 3.17. Excision biopsy specimen after prior vacuum-assisted biopsy

3.3 Overview of Biopsy Techniques

As indicated on the previous pages, there are several methods available to biopsy breast tissue (Figs. 3.18a–d, 3.19a–d, 3.20). The optimal method depends on the amount of tissue required and the objective of the biopsy (whether to completely excise a breast lesion or simply obtain a sample) (Fig. 3.19a–d). The greatest amount of tissue is obtained with open biopsy techniques (excisional biopsy or needle-localized biopsy; Fig. 3.19a), and decreasing amounts are obtained by biopsy with the advanced breast biopsy instrument (ABBI) system (Fig. 3.19b), core biopsy (Fig. 3.19c), and vacuum-assisted biopsy (Figs. 3.8, 3.9, 3.10, 3.19d). The more tissue required, the greater the size of the incision required for the procedure. Thus, a very small incision is required for vacuum-assisted biopsy, and increasingly larger incisions are required for the core biopsy, ABBI system, and open biopsy methods.

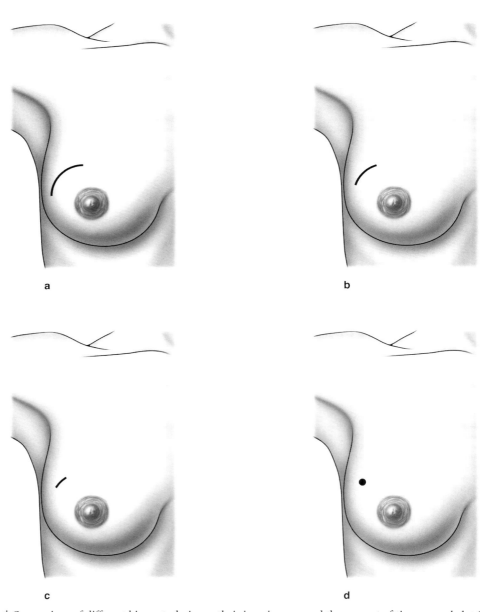

a

b

c

d

Fig. 3.18a–d. Comparison of different biopsy techniques, their invasiveness, and the amount of tissue sampled. a Excisional or needle-localized biopsy; b the advanced breast biopsy instrument (*ABBI*) system; c core biopsy; d the stereotactic vacuum-assisted biopsy device

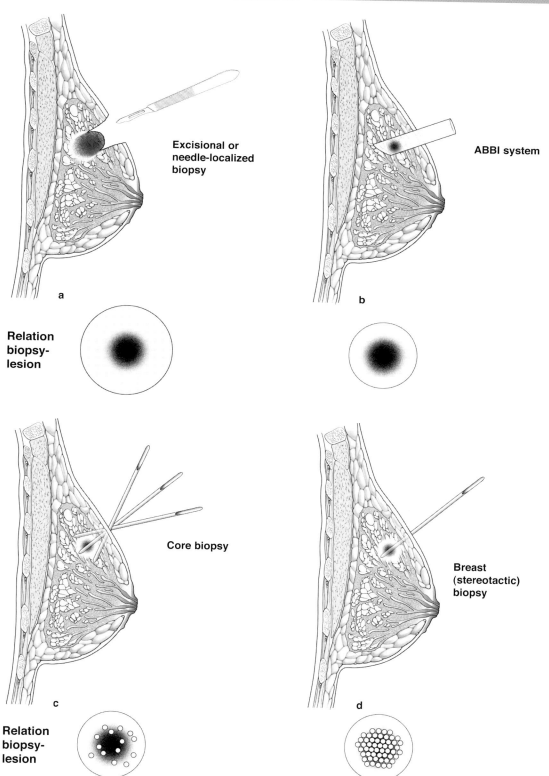

Fig. 3.19a–d. Comparison of different biopsy techniques, their invasiveness, and the amount of tissue sampled. a Excisional or needle-localized biopsy; b the advanced breast biopsy instrument (*ABBI*) system; c core biopsy; d the stereotactic vacuum-assisted biopsy device

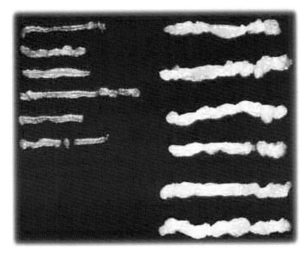

Fig. 3.20. Examples of core-cut (*left*) and vacuum-assisted (*right*) specimens

3.4 Needle-Localized Biopsy

A needle-localized biopsy (Fig. 3.21) is performed to assess abnormalities of the breast that are not palpable but are seen on mammogram. To obtain tissue for histological evaluation, the surgeon requires the assistance of the radiologist to localize the mammographic abnormality with a hooked wire.

The patient is first transported to the radiology suite, where the mammographic abnormality is localized with a hooked wire (Fig. 3.22). Proper placement of the wire within the abnormality is essential. Mammograms with two views (anterior–posterior and medio–lateral) should be obtained showing the wire and its relationship to the abnormality. These mammograms guide the surgeon during dissection.

The patient is transported to the operating room with the wire in place. Care should be taken to ensure that the wire is secured on the surface of the breast during transport. The outer part of the wire should be carefully taped on the surface of the breast.

The needle-localized biopsy can be performed using either local or general anesthetic, depending on preferences of the patient and surgeon. The tape is carefully removed from the wire and surface of the breast, and a wide area of the breast is cleaned with a sterilizing solution. A curvilinear incision is made immediately adjacent to the wire, along the direction of one of the natural skin crease lines (lines of Langer). Hooks are used to lift up the edges of the skin. With the needle-localized mammograms serving as a guide, the wire and tissue around it is removed en bloc by sharp dissection. Electrocautery should be avoided during dissection, as this can create artifacts that obscure pathological assessment of the specimen. However, once the wire and breast tissue around it are removed, meticulous attention is paid to achieving hemostasis with electrocautery.

It should be emphasized that the incision should be placed near the wire. Periareolar incisions and inframammary incisions are not recommended, unless the wire is immediately adjacent to these areas (Fig. 3.23, 3.24).

Once the breast tissue (with the wire in it) is removed, the specimen is transported to the radiology suite. A specimen film is obtained to confirm excision of the mammographic abnormality. After this is done, the breast wound is irrigated, and skin edges are re-approximated using a running absorbable subcuticular stitch.

Figure 3.22a–c shows: (1) a mammographic abnormality with a wire localizing it (medio-lateral view); (2) a mammographic abnormality with a wire localizing it (craniocaudal view); and (3) a specimen film of the completely excised mammographic abnormality with the wire through it.

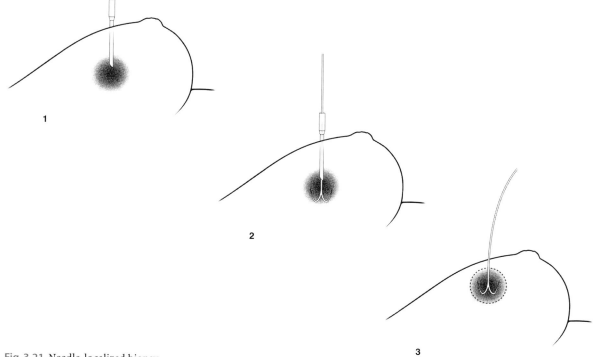

Fig. 3.21. Needle-localized biopsy

3

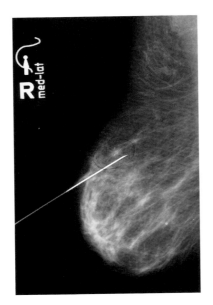

a

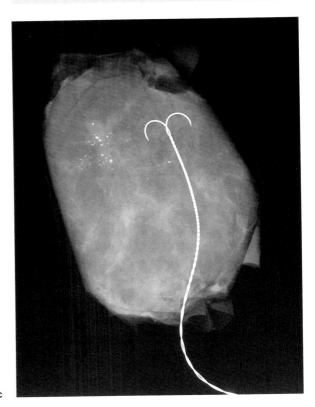

c

b

Fig. 3.22a, b Mammogram of the right breast. c Radiograph of the breast tissue specimen with microcalcifications (magnification 2 fold)

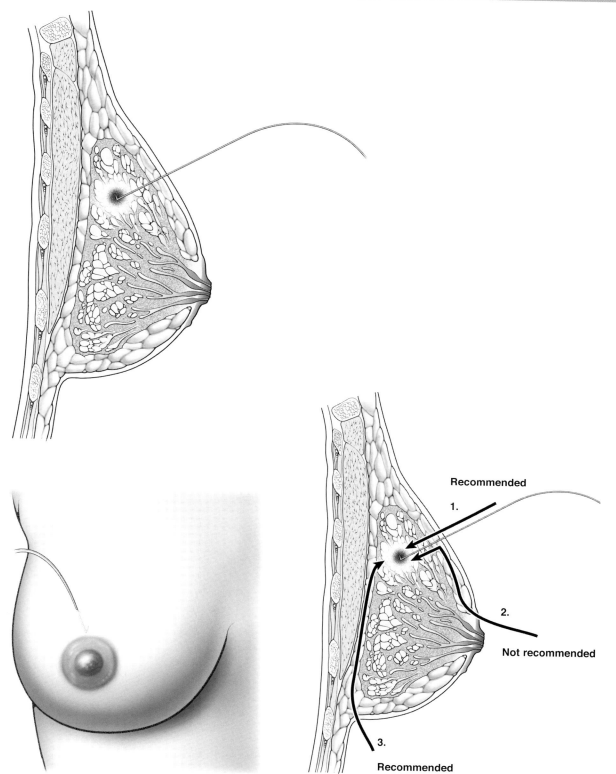

Fig. 3.23. Guidance for correct approach during needle-localized biopsy. The posterior glandular approach (*1* on *right*) is recommended, whereas periareolar (*2* on *right*) is not recommended. Inframammary approach (*3 on right*) is only recommended if the tumor is deeply located

3

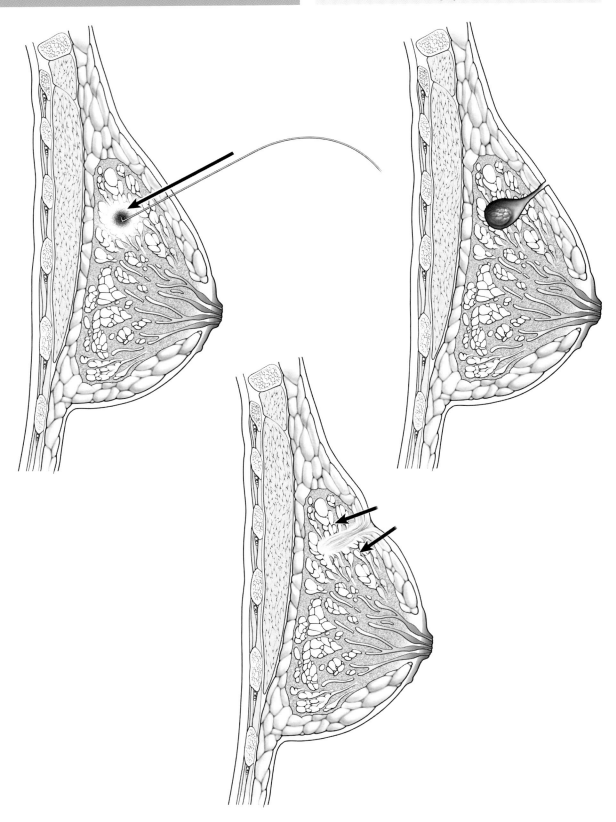

Fig. 3.24. Needle-localized biopsy

3.5 Microductectomy

This technique is used to excise a single breast duct, usually to diagnose the cause of nipple discharge from a single duct. If bloody nipple discharge arises from a single duct, it is often attributable to a papilloma.

Surgical procedures around the nipple–areola complex are uncomfortable for the patient, and many surgeons prefer to use a general anesthetic. A catheter attached to a thin butterfly syringe is used to instill blue-dye into the lactiferous duct and sinus (Fig. 3.25a, b). The catheter is removed, and a periareolar incision made. Tissues are dissected down to the duct containing the blue-dye. The duct is excised and submitted for pathological evaluation. Afterwards, meticulous attention should be paid to achieving hemostasis with electrocautery. The wound is then irrigated, and the skin edges re-approximated with a running subcuticular absorbable stitch.

Alternatively, a periareolar incision can be made and the areolar lifted up with a skin hook (Fig. 3.26). The area of breast tissue that includes the involved duct (or ducts) is broadly excised, extending the area of excision posteriorly. Once the tissue is excised and hemostasis is obtained, the posterior extent of the excision within the breast can be re-approximated with interrupted absorbable stitches, and the nipple–areola complex re-attached to the adjacent skin with a running 3–0 Monocryl subcuticular stitch.

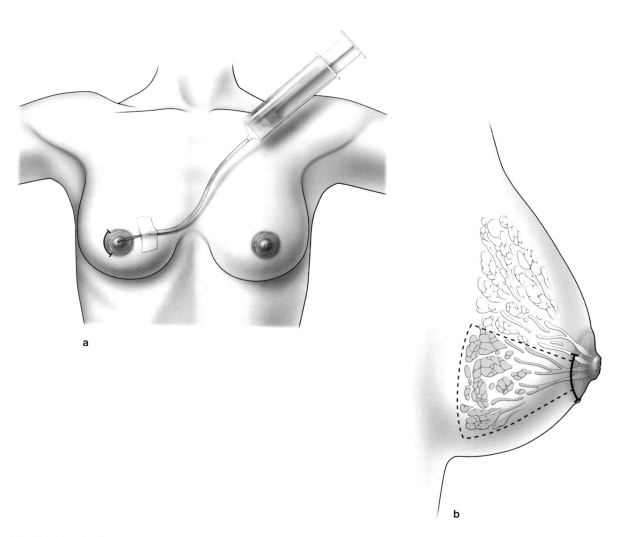

Fig. 3.25a, b. Microductectomy. a Blue-dye is injected into the lactiferous duct and sinus using a thin butterfly syringe. b Tissue stained by the blue-dye is removed (*dotted line*)

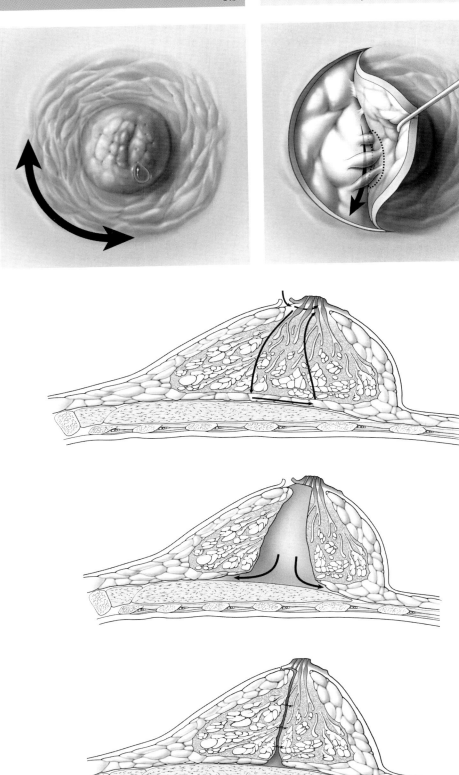

Fig. 3.26. Ductectomy through a periareolar incision

3.6 Subareolar Dissection

A subareolar dissection is required to extirpate the major ducts immediately below their opening at the nipple (Fig. 3.27). This procedure is often used to diagnose or treat persistent nipple discharge (usually unilateral) arising from many ducts. In many cases, such discharge is attributable to duct ectasia. However, there are other causes of profuse nipple discharge involving many ducts, particularly if the discharge is bilateral, including a prolactin-secreting tumor. Therefore, patients must undergo thorough assessment prior to surgery.

This procedure is usually performed under a general anesthetic. After applying a sterilizing solution over the entire field, a periareolar incision is made, and the major duct system immediately below the nipple–areola complex is excised. Meticulous attention is paid to hemostasis using electrocautery. The wound is copiously irrigated, and the skin edges are re-approximated with a running absorbable subcuticular stitch.

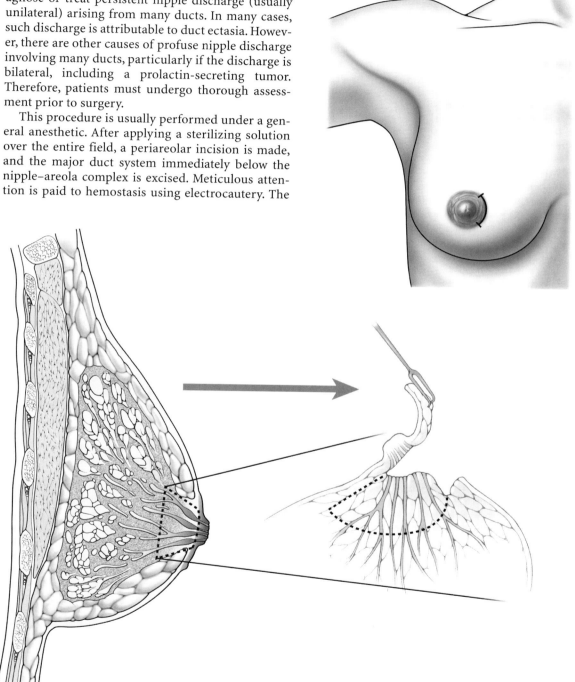

Fig. 3.27. Subareolar dissection, required to extirpate the major ducts immediately below the nipple

3.7 Mammary Ductoscopy

Figures 3.28–3.34 are courtesy of Professor Kefah Mokbel, London, UK.

Mammary ductoscopy is relatively new technology and its potential applications are still under investigation. However, it has been used to diagnose the source of discharge from a single breast duct (Fig. 3.28). The orifice of the breast duct is dilated, and a small endoscope is passed through it into the ductal system. The small endoscope contains a camera, and this allows for direct visualization of the intraductal system on a television screen. Thus, intraductal pathology can be visualized, allowing for adequate removal of intraductal lesions while preserving surrounding normal breast tissue.

The ductoscopes that are now frequently used are 1.0 mm in external diameter with a 0.45 mm working channel (Fig. 3.29), allowing air insufflation and saline irrigation during visualization. The working channel provides for ductal dilatation, sampling of intraductal lesions, and also permits irrigation of debris, thereby providing a clear image (Fig. 3.30). Ductoscopes have been utilized in the management of nipple discharge, to help determine the underlying cause of the discharge. Additionally, lavage of the ductal system through the ductoscope (ductal lavage) is under investigation as a means of harvesting epithelial cells, examining these cells for evidence of atypia or malignancy (Figs. 3.31, 3.32, 3.33 and 3.34), and thereby assessing women at high risk for developing breast cancer.

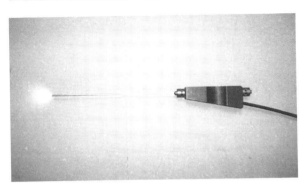

Fig. 3.29. The endoscope, which has an external diameter of 1 mm, a 0.45-mm working channel and a resolution of 10,000 pixels

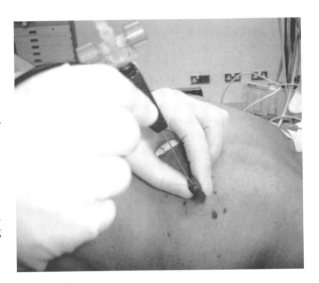

Fig. 3.30. The procedure

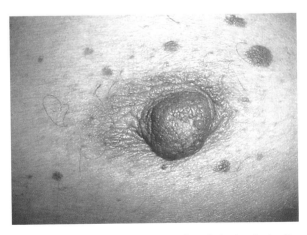

Fig. 3.28. Mammary ductoscopy and pathologic nipple discharge (PND)

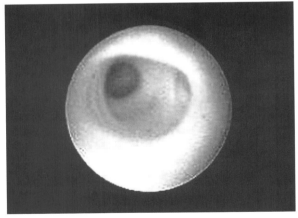

Fig. 3.31. Normal mammary duct visualized on ductoscopy

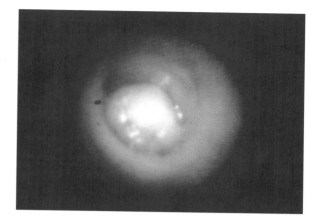

Fig. 3.32. Papilloma visualized on ductoscopy

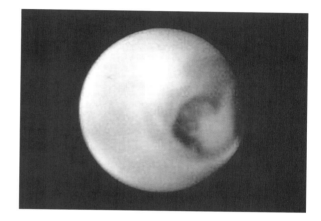

Fig. 3.33. Ductal carcinoma in situ (*DCIS*) visualized on ductoscopy

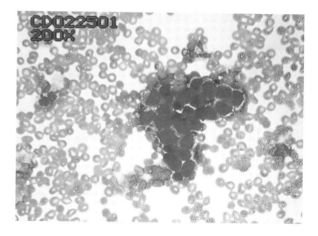

Fig. 3.34. Ductoscopic cytology (DCIS)

Chapter 4

Surgery for Benign Breast Diseases

4.1 Cyst Aspiration

The technique used to aspirate a palpable breast cyst is similar to that used for fine needle aspiration cytology (Fig. 3.2). The skin surface is cleansed with rubbing alcohol. We generally attach a 21-gauge needle attached to a 20-ml syringe. The cyst is secured with the thumb and index fingers or the index and middle fingers. The syringe is held with the other hand, and the cyst aspirated until it is no longer palpable. The contents of a cyst generally contain brown, yellow, or greenish fluid. If such fluid is obtained on aspiration, then there is no need to send it for cytological evaluation. Cytology is necessary only if bloody fluid is obtained on aspiration.

If a cyst is noted on ultrasound but is not palpable, then ultrasound-guided needle aspiration might be indicated. Again, the skin surface is cleansed with rubbing alcohol. The ultrasound probe is held with one hand, identifying the cyst. The syringe is held with the other hand, and the cyst aspirated. Figure 4.1 also shows a cyst aspiration under ultrasound guidance. The cyst is seen in the upper panel (Fig. 4.1a) ultrasound view, and a needle though the cyst is seen in the lower panel (Fig. 4.1b) ultrasound view.

4

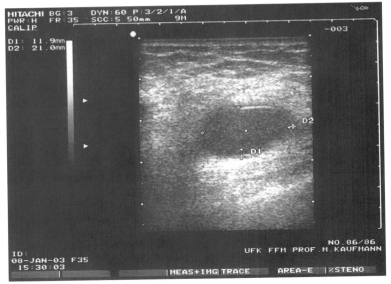

a

b

Fig. 4.1a, b. Cyst aspiration under ultrasound guidance

4.2 Excision of Intraductal Papilloma

The galactography in Fig. 4.2 depicts an intraductal papilloma, the most common cause of bloody nipple discharge arising from a single duct. Generally, these patients are managed conservatively, the papilloma sloughs off, and the bloody discharge usually resolves spontaneously over a period of several weeks. If this does not occur, then excision of the involved duct might be indicated. The procedure for excision of a breast duct is described in Chap. 3.

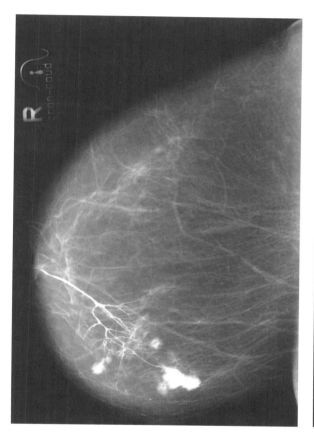
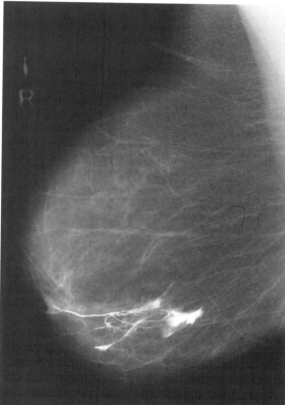

Fig. 4.2. Galactography of an intraductal papilloma

4.3 Excision of Giant Fibroadenoma

Fibroadenomas are benign lesions, generally found in younger women. The clinical examination may lead a physician to suspect a fibroadenoma in a young woman who presents with a palpable breast mass. These lesions are hard, well circumscribed, and mobile. On palpation, a fibroadenoma may resemble a marble rolling under the fingertips. However, the definitive diagnosis of fibroadenoma is often only established after excisional biopsy. In a young woman with a suspected fibroadenoma, an excisional biopsy should be performed, if possible through a periareolar incision. This results in the best cosmetic outcome.

If a patient presents with a giant fibroadenoma, the fibroadenoma is translocated to the site of the nipple–areola complex with the surgeon's nondominant hand. Then, with the dominant hand, the surgeon places a periareolar or inframammary incision directly over the fibroadenoma, and the lesion is excised through this incision (Fig. 4.3). The fibroadenoma is excised using sharp dissection, staying close to the edge of the lesion. After the fibroadenoma is removed, meticulous attention should be paid to hemostasis, using electrocautery. The wound is then copiously irrigated and we generally approximate the skin edges with a running 3-0 or 4-0 Monocryl subcuticular stitch.

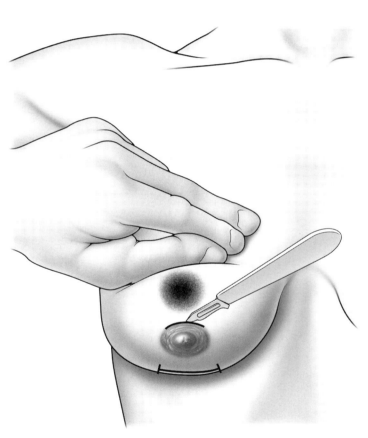

Fig. 4.3. Excision of giant fibroadenoma (periareolar or alternative inframammary incision)

4.4 Drainage of a Breast Abscess

If a patient presents with an area on the breast that is erythematous, warm, and fluctuant, this generally indicates the presence of an underlying abscess. An abscess of the breast should be drained emergently. In most instances, a breast abscess is drained in a manner identical to drainage of an abscess anywhere else. That is, an incision is made directly over the abscess cavity, the pus drained out, and the wound packed open. However, there are some techniques that can be applied specifically to the drainage of a breast abscess. These techniques may minimize unnecessary scarring, and result in a better appearance of the breast postoperatively.

As indicated in Fig. 4.4, some large abscesses can be drained through a periareolar incision, placing a Penrose drain through the abscess. The drain can be brought out through the inframammary fold. A safety pin is attached to prevent the drain from dislodging. The drain is kept in place for several days, until drainage subsides.

Alternatively, an abscess can be drained through a periareolar incision, and the wound dissected bluntly until the abscess cavity is reached and the pus drains out (Fig. 4.5). The wound should be packed open with a strip of gauze. Patients should be taught to change the dressings on a daily basis until the wound granulates and closes.

If a patient presents with a subareolar abscess, a lacrimal duct probe can be placed into the abscess cavity and brought out through the affected breast duct on the surface of the nipple, as illustrated (Fig. 4.6).

Large abscess cavities on the posterior aspect of the breast are sometimes drained through an incision in the inframammary fold, placing a drainage catheter into the abscess cavity (Fig. 4.7). The placement of the catheter sometimes requires ultrasound guidance.

It should be emphasized that erythema of the breast can be attributable to an underlying abscess, cellulitis, or inflammatory breast cancer. To exclude the possibility of an inflammatory breast cancer, a full thickness biopsy of the skin is sometimes indicated. Thus, any patient who presents with breast erythema must undergo thorough evaluation.

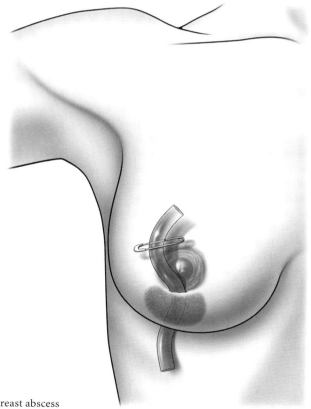

Fig. 4.4. Drainage of a larger breast abscess

4

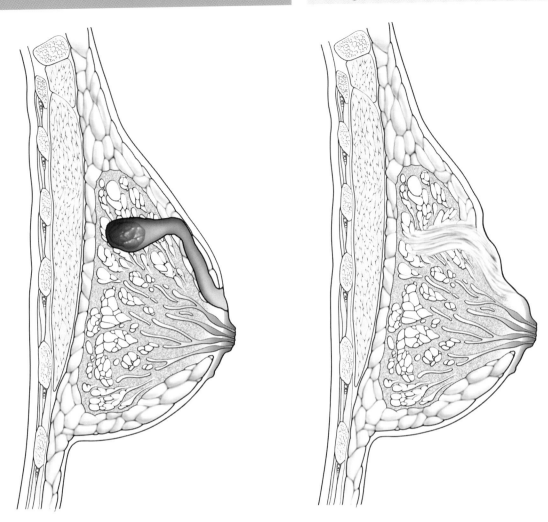

Fig. 4.5. Drainage of a large abscess through a periareolar incision

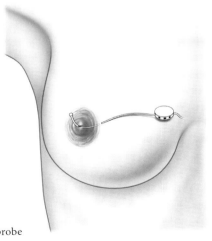

Fig. 4.6. Drainage of a subareolar abscess using a lacrimal duct probe

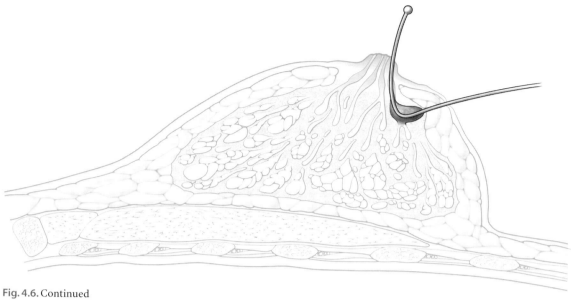

Fig. 4.6. Continued

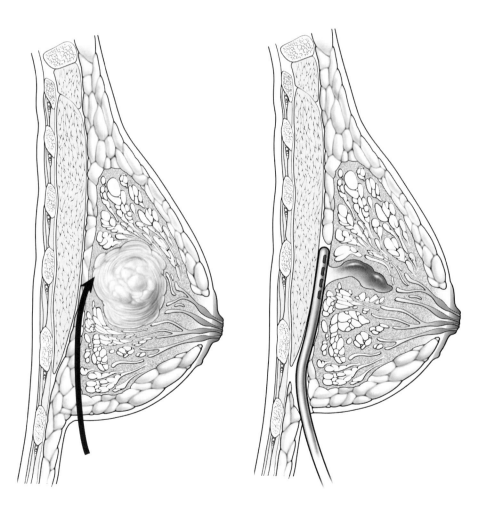

Fig. 4.7. Drainage of an abscess through an incision located in the sulcus

4.5 Surgical Management of Gynecomastia

Gynecomastia refers to hypertrophy of the breast tissue in males. The area of hypertrophy is generally immediately beneath the nipple–areola complex. As illustrated in the accompanying diagrams, there are several methods to treat gynecomastia.

One option is to make a periareolar incision (Fig. 4.8a). This incision can be extended further laterally and medially, as illustrated. The nipple–areola complex is then retracted anteriorly, and the underlying breast tissue is extirpated either by sharp dissection or liposuction. Afterwards, hemostasis is achieved using electrocautery, the wound is copiously irrigated, and skin edges are re-approximated with a running 3–0 or 4–0 Monocryl subcuticular stitch.

An alternate approach is to use the round block incision (Fig. 4.8b). In this technique, an area around the nipple–areolar complex is de-epithelialized. Again, the glandular tissue can be removed either by sharp dissection or liposuction, directly through this area of de-epithelialization. Hemostasis is achieved with electrocautery and the skin edges are re-approximated with running 3–0 or 4–0 Monocryl subcuticular stitches.

Yet another technique utilizes a W incision within the areolar, avoiding the nipple itself (Fig. 4.8c). The tissue along the lines of the incision will retract away, and the surgeon excises the underlying tissue. After achieving hemostasis, the skin edges are re-approximated with absorbable stitches.

No matter which technique is used, a large area of breast tissue can be excised beneath the nipple–areola complex (Fig. 4.8d).

The gynecomastia can be treated with liposuction (Fig. 4.9a, b). The liposuction can be introduced either through a periareolar incision (Fig. 4.9c, d) or through a round block incision (Fig. 4.9e, f).

For a man with a markedly enlarged breast, the gynecomastia is often best treated with a subcutaneous mastectomy (Fig. 4.10). This can be done through a periareolar incision or through an incision along the inframammary fold. The entire breast is removed, leaving a small rim of tissue immediately beneath the nipple–areola complex. The surgeon should also be careful to leave a rim of breast tissue under the skin, so that blood supply to the skin is preserved. Through a separate stab incision inferiorly, a Jackson–Pratt drain is brought out and tied in place with 3–0 nylon stitch. This drain can be removed in a few days, once drainage subsides.

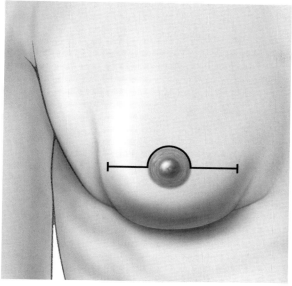

a

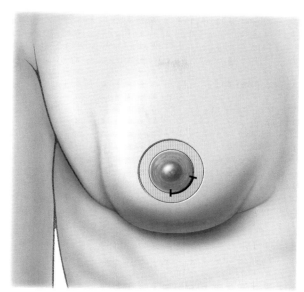

b

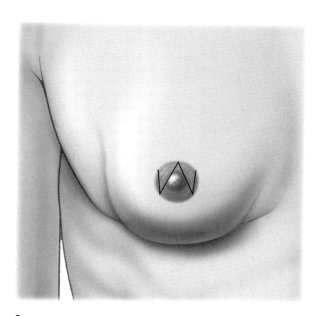

c

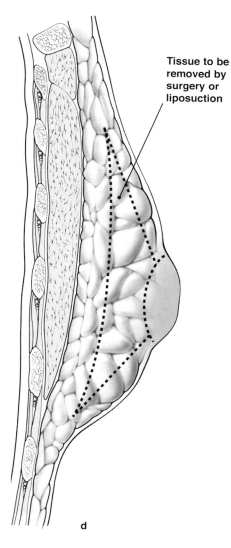

Tissue to be removed by surgery or liposuction

d

Fig. 4.8a–d. Surgical management of gynecomastia.
a Nipple–areola complex incision.
b Round block incision and de-epithelialization periareolar.
c "W" incision.
d To show the area of breast tissue excised beneath the nipple–areola complex

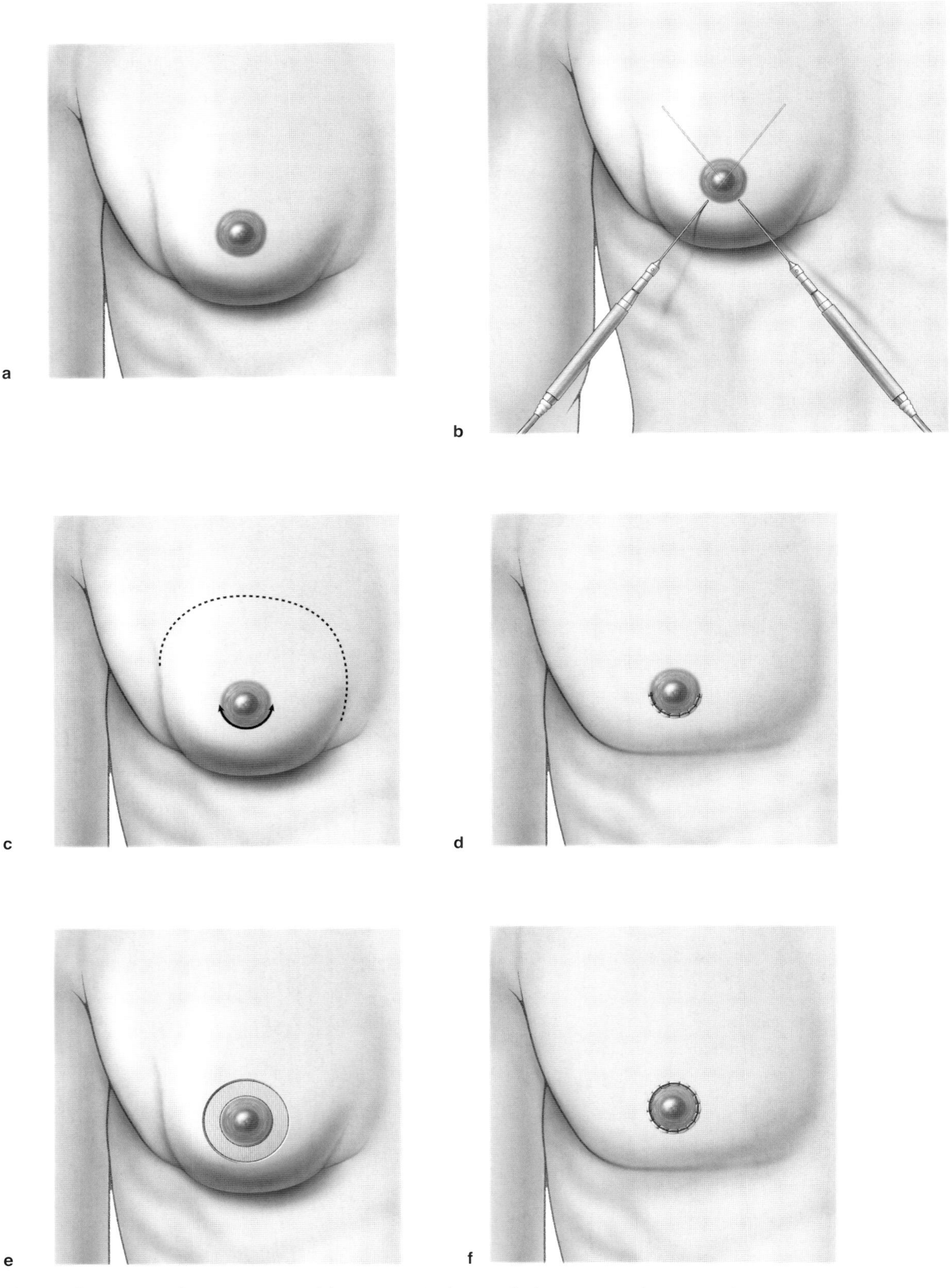

4

Fig. 4.9a–f. Treatment of gynecomastia with liposuction. (Indication for liposuction only in cases of fatty tissue or in addition for body conturing)

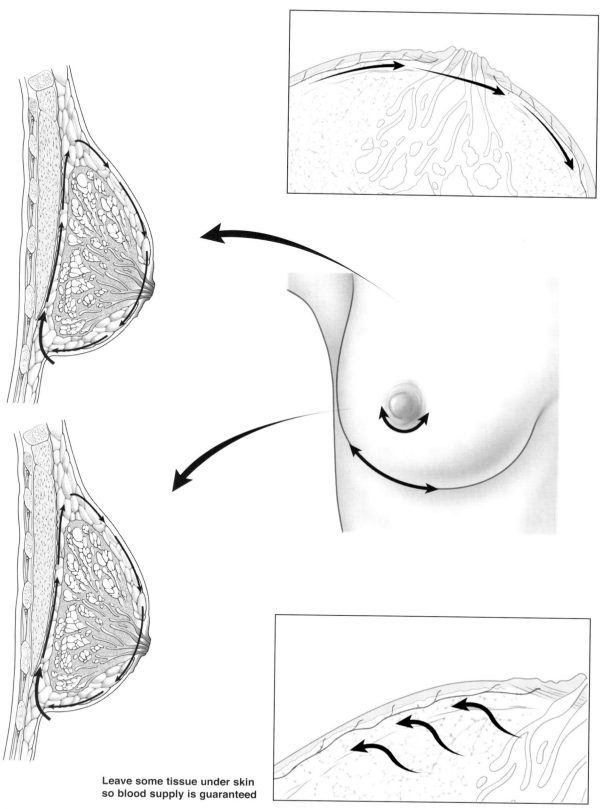

**Leave some tissue under skin
so blood supply is guaranteed**

Fig. 4.10. Treatment of gynecomastia with subcutaneous mastectomy

Chapter 5

Biopsy Procedures

5.1 Incision Lines for Excisional Biopsy

Excisional biopsy refers to the complete extirpation of a breast mass. The objective is to remove the entire breast mass with a minimal amount of normal tissue around it. An excisional biopsy is sometimes performed to establish a diagnosis. If, following excisional biopsy, the mass proves to be malignant and pathological assessment reveals that margins are free of tumor, then extirpation of additional breast tissue is generally not necessary. In most instances, such patients will require radiotherapy. An excisional biopsy is sometimes referred to as a lumpectomy or wide excision.

It is important to remember that natural lines of skin tension, known as Langer lines, extend outwards circumferentially from the nipple–areola complex. Therefore, at or above the level of the nipple, when performing an excisional biopsy, the incision should never be placed perpendicular to the natural lines of skin tension (Figs. 5.1, 5.2). Rather, the incision should follow these lines and be placed in a semicircular or periareolar fashion.

Below the nipple, the incision lines may be placed radially or along the inframammary fold, as illustrated (Fig. 5.1, 5.2.1, 5.2.2).

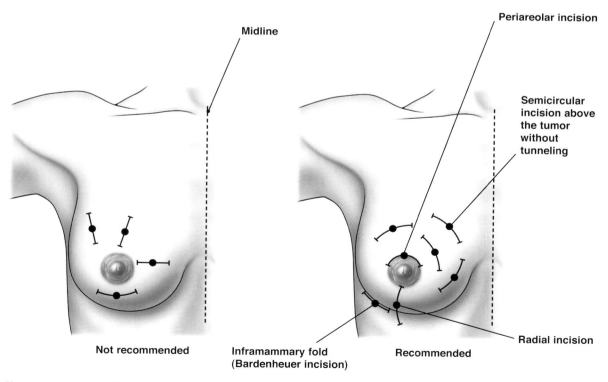

Fig. 5.1. Recommended incision lines for excisional biopsy

5

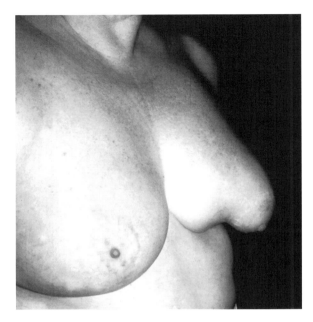

Fig. 5.2.1. Semicircular incision in the lower quadrant for breast-conserving surgery is not recommended

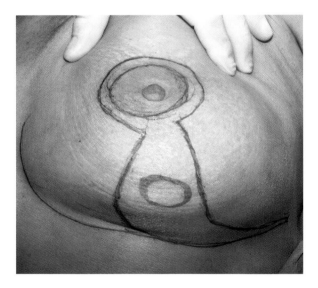

Fig. 5.2.2. Radial incision in the lower quadrant for breast-conserving surgery is recommended ("B-technique")

5.2 Variants of Incisions and Extent of Breast Cancer Surgery

In the late nineteenth century, William Halsted promulgated radical mastectomy as the optimal treatment for primary breast cancer. This operation involves removal of the breast, underlying pectoralis muscle, and ipsilateral axillary lymph nodes. The incision for this procedure, illustrated in Fig. 5.3a, incorporates both the breast and axilla. This is a disfiguring procedure, and generally no longer recommended in the treatment of primary breast cancer.

The modified radical mastectomy is less disfiguring because the pectoralis muscles are spared. The modified radical mastectomy removes the breast and adjacent axillary lymph nodes. As illustrated in the accompanying diagram, an elliptical incision (Stewart incision) is generally used, incorporating the breast and extending to the axilla (Fig. 5.3b). It is important to note that the incision also incorporates the primary tumor. Both the breast and adjacent axillary contents are removed through this incision. Many surgeons recommend the modified radical mastectomy for treating patients with very large primary tumors or multicentric tumors (tumors in more than one quadrant of the breast).

The aim of the skin-sparing mastectomy is to remove the entire breast and yet preserve as much skin as possible over the breast, to facilitate reconstructive surgery. Therefore, a narrow elliptical incision is made that incorporates the nipple–areola complex, but not necessarily the primary breast tumor (Fig. 5.3c). Skin flaps are raised, and the entire breast, including the tumor, is extirpated. The axillary contents are removed by extending the mastectomy incision to the axilla.

Six large, randomized prospective trials have shown that the extent of mastectomy has no impact on breast cancer mortality. Yet, the extent of mastectomy does influence the risk of local recurrence. Therefore, patients who undergo less extensive mastectomies (breast-conserving surgery) generally require radiotherapy to reduce the risk of local recurrence. Breast-conserving surgery is now widely accepted as the standard treatment for breast cancer. Two separate incisions are required: one to remove the primary breast tumor, and the other to remove the axillary contents. When performing breast-conserving surgery, there are various forms of incisions that can be made to remove the primary breast tumor, and these are illustrated. Quadrantectomy (Fig. 5.3d) involves removal of the entire quadrant of the breast containing the tumor, and this is done through a curvilinear incision, as illustrated. A segmental excision or lumpectomy (Fig. 5.3e) is performed using a curvilinear incision along a natural skin crease (line of Langer), placed over the tumor. Once this incision is made, skin flaps are raised, and the underlying tumor with a segment of normal tissue is extirpated. The incision should be made directly over the tumor, and the entire tumor with a margin of normal tissue is extirpated. A new approach of nipple sparing mastectomy is currently tested at the European Institute of Oncology (Milan), allowing the preservation of the nipple areola complex for cancer requiring a mastectomy. Prevention of local recurrence behind the areola is performed with an intraoperative radiotherapy.

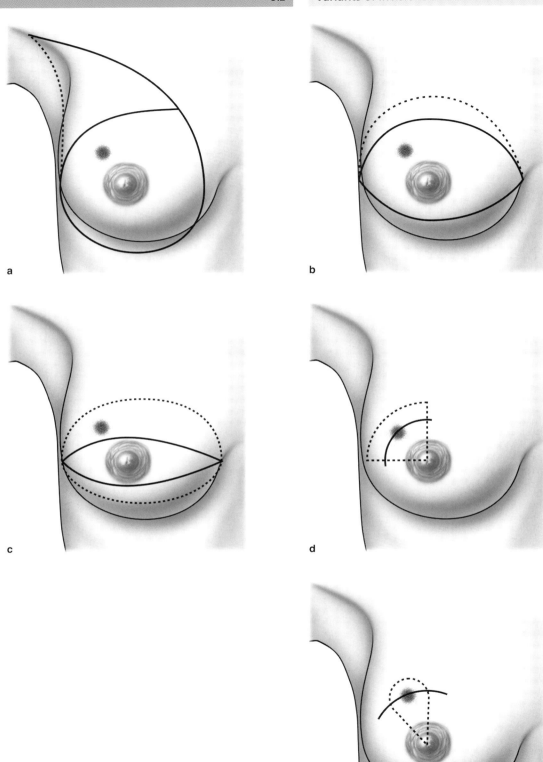

a

b

c

d

e

Fig. 5.3a–e. Variants of incisions and extent
of breast cancer surgery

5.3 Lumpectomy (Wide Excision)

As indicated previously, an excisional biopsy is performed with a curvilinear incision along a natural skin crease line (line of Langer) (Fig. 5.4). If the tumor is close to the skin, an elliptical incision is made (Fig. 5.5), and the skin within the ellipse is included with the specimen.

Once the incision is made, sharp dissection is used to remove the tumor with a margin of healthy tissue around it. Two fingers are used to identify the tumor, and healthy tissue around it is sharply divided using scissors (Fig. 5.4). It is preferable not to use electrocautery during dissection, as this may create artifacts, making it difficult for the pathologist to evaluate surgical margins. However, once the tumor is removed, electrocautery must be meticulously applied to achieve hemostasis. The most common complication following lumpectomy is a postoperative hematoma. After hemostasis is achieved, the wound is copiously irrigated and skin edges are re-approximated with a running absorbable subcuticular stitch. We prefer to use 3–0 Monocryl for this purpose.

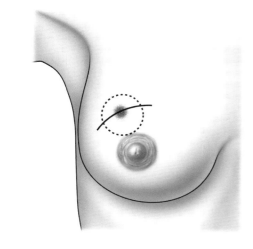

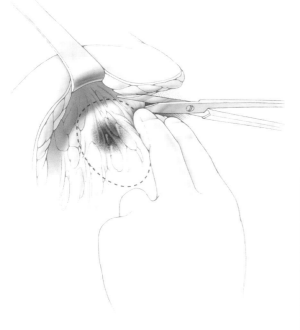

Fig. 5.4. Lumpectomy (wide excision). Resection outlines within healthy margins identified by two fingers

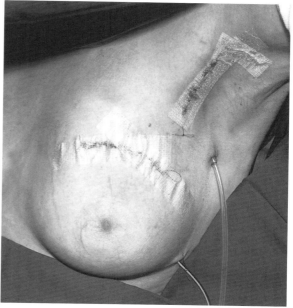

Fig. 5.5. Recommended: semicircular incision in the upper quadrant over the tumor and separate incision in the axilla

5

5.4 Specimen Management for the Pathologist

Once the specimen is removed, the surgeon should inspect and palpate it to make certain that there is no evidence of gross tumor at the margins. The surgeon must appropriately orient the specimen before submitting it to the pathologist (Fig. 5.6). Thus, the pathologist must be made aware of the anterior, posterior, superior, inferior, medial, and lateral margins.

This is essential for appropriate pathological evaluation. If margins are not free of tumor, the pathologist must inform the surgeon which margins are involved.

There are two ways to orient the specimen for the pathologist. One method is to apply colored ink to differentiate the various surfaces of the specimen. Another method is to use stitches to orient the specimen. For example, two long stitches might be placed on the lateral surface, one long stitch on the anterior surface, two short stitches on the inferior surface, etc.

If the margins of the specimen are involved with tumor, the patient may require further excision of the biopsy cavity. However, if the margins are free of tumor, then there is generally no need to re-excise the biopsy cavity. As mentioned previously, most of these patients will receive radiotherapy.

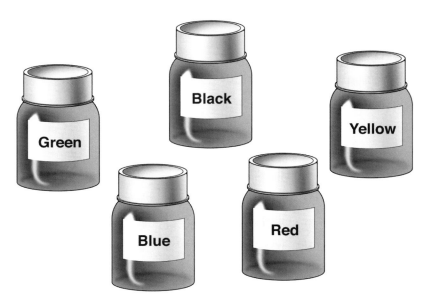

Fig. 5.6. Specimen management for the pathologist

Chapter 6

Surgery for Breast Carcinoma

6.1 Modified Radical Mastectomy

In evaluating a patient for mastectomy, the location of the tumor is of critical importance. When referring to the location of a tumor in the breast, keep in mind that the breast is divided into four quadrants: upper outer, upper inner, lower outer, and lower inner. The location of the tumor determines the type of incision required for the mastectomy. In general, an elliptical incision is made, incorporating the nipple–areola complex, and extending towards the axilla (Fig. 6.1). It should be emphasized that the term "modified radical mastectomy" refers to removal of the entire breast and extirpation of the adjacent lymph nodes in the axilla. The pectoralis major and minor muscles are preserved. In contrast, the term "simple mastectomy" refers to the extirpation of the breast alone, without extirpation of the axillary lymph nodes. In the simple mastectomy, the pectoralis major and minor muscles are preserved as well. The incision for the simple mastectomy is depicted in the accompanying illustration (Fig. 6.2).

The following figures demonstrate various incisions for patients undergoing modified radical mastectomy. The type of incision required depends on the location of the primary tumor in the breast.

For tumors in the upper outer quadrant of the breast, the incision should extend around the nipple–areola complex, the tumor, and into the axilla, as illustrated in the accompanying diagram (Fig. 6.3a). Upper outer quadrant tumors are most common, and this diagram (Fig. 6.3b) illustrates the most common incision for mastectomy.

For tumors in the upper inner quadrant, the incision again incorporates the tumor and the nipple–areola complex, extending to the axilla (Fig. 6.4a). However, as shown in the accompanying diagram (Fig. 6.4b), the final incision, when approximated, may actually show two scars perpendicular to one another.

If the tumor is in the lower outer quadrant of the breast, a triangular incision might be required, extending around the tumor and nipple–areola complex, with the lateral extent of the incision oriented towards the axilla (Fig. 6.5a). The final scar may resemble a U, as shown in the accompanying diagram (Fig. 6.5b).

For tumors in the lower inner quadrant, the incision incorporates both the tumor and the nipple–areola complex, with the lateral extent of the incision extending towards the axilla (Fig. 6.6a). The final incision, when approximated, may show two scars perpendicular to one another, as indicated in the accompanying diagram (Fig. 6.6b).

It is important to emphasize that, for all these tumors, the lateral extent of the incisions should extend towards the axilla, because both the mastectomy and axillary dissections are carried out through the same incision.

When performing a mastectomy, the surgeon should pay careful attention to the thickness of the skin flaps. Although the breast tissue must be removed, ample subcutaneous tissue must be preserved, so that blood perfusion to the skin is not compromised.

The skin incision should be made incorporating both the tumor and nipple–areola complex, as illustrated previously. The assistant should lift the skin with hooks, applying vertical traction. The surgeon applies counter-traction inferiorly on the breast with one hand, leaving the other hand free to perform the dissection. The surgeon should identify a plane of tissue between the breast and the subcutaneous tissue that is relatively avascular, and dissect this sharply. We prefer to use a knife for this dissection, although some surgeons use electrocautery. If the surgeon encounters any bleeding during the dissection, hemostasis is achieved with electrocautery. The dissection should proceed superiorly to about the level of the clavicle, inferiorly to the level of the rectus abdominis muscle, medially to the sternum, and laterally to the latissimus dorsi muscle. Once the anterior surface of the breast is dissected free from the overlying subcutaneous tissue, then its posterior surface should be dissected free from the underlying pectoralis major muscle using electrocautery. Fig. 6.6.1a–f demonstrates how to close the defect of an extensive mastectomy ("suspension technique").

Once the mastectomy is completed, the surgeon proceeds with an axillary dissection, and this technique is illustrated later in the text when we discuss the breast-conserving surgery techniques. It should be emphasized that, in the modified radical mastectomy, the breast and axillary contents are generally extirpated as a single specimen. At the end of the procedure, a Jackson–Pratt drain is brought out through a separate stab incision in the axilla and sewn in place with 2–0 or 3–0 nylon. We close the wound by placing interrupted 3–0 Dexon stitches subcutaneously, with a running 3–0 Monocryl subcuticular stitch to re-approximate the skin edges.

6

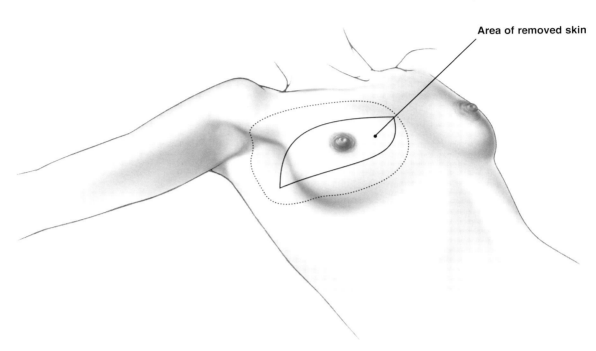

Area of removed skin

Fig. 6.1. Incision for modified radical (Patey) mastectomy

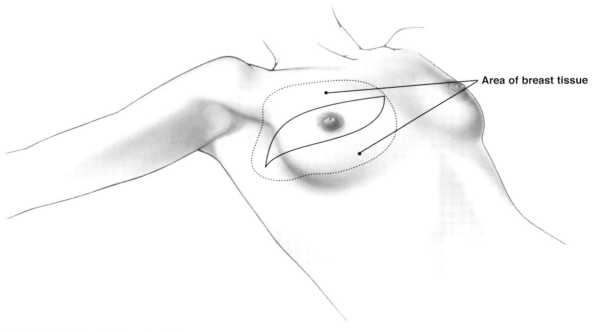

Area of breast tissue

Fig. 6.2. Incision for simple mastectomy

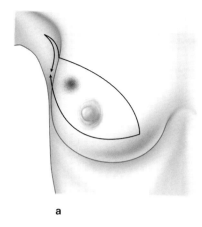

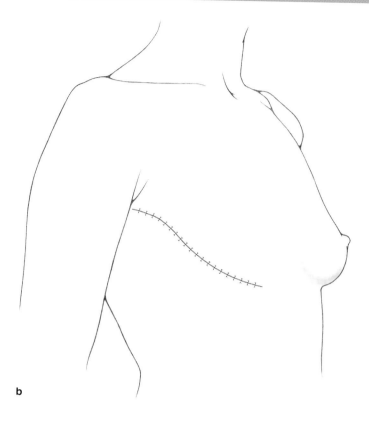

Fig. 6.3a, b. Mastectomy: type of incision for a tumor in the upper outer quadrant

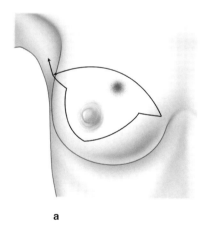

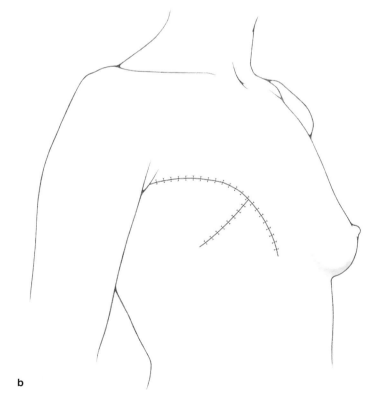

Fig. 6.4a, b. Mastectomy: type of incision for a tumor in the upper inner quadrant

6

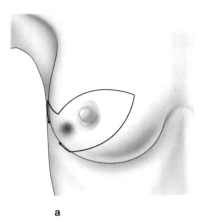

a

b

Fig. 6.5a, b. Mastectomy: type of incision
for a tumor in the inferior outer quadrant

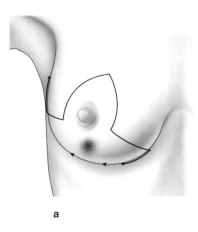

a

b

Fig. 6.6a, b. Mastectomy: type of incision
for a tumor in the inferior quadrant

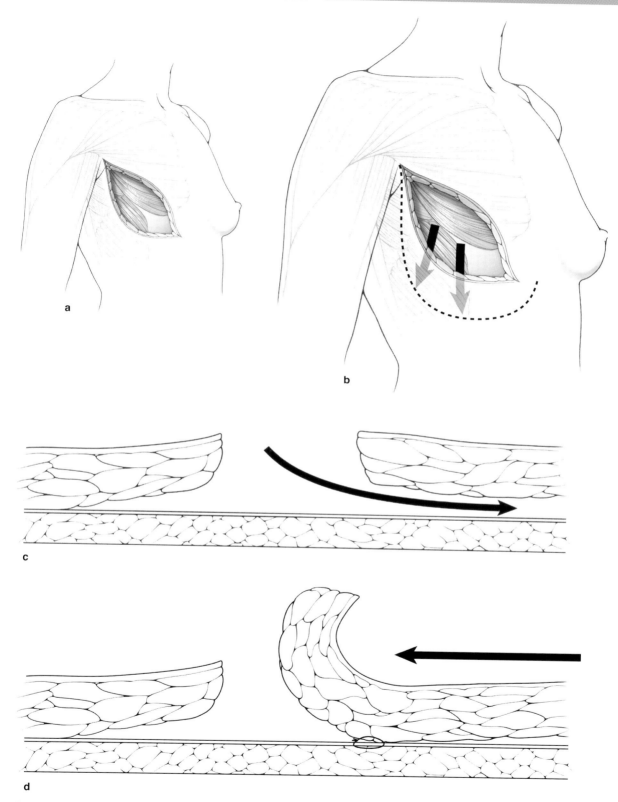

Fig. 6.6.1a–f. Closure of defect of an extensive mastectomy without tension on the skin. This is also used for immediate breast reconstruction using the "suspension technique," mobilizing tissue to accommodate the prosthesis (see Chapter 7)

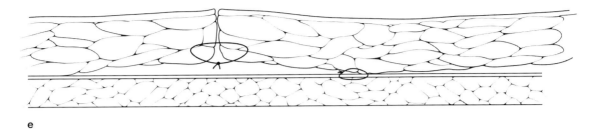

e

6

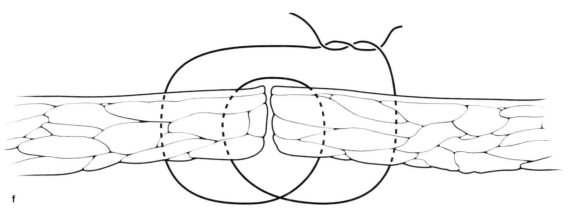

f

Fig. 6.6.1a–f. Continued

6.2 Simple Mastectomy

Simple mastectomy refers to removal of only the breast, with no dissection of the axilla. It is often followed by immediate breast reconstruction, and this is discussed later in this text (Chap. 7). There are several possible reasons why a surgeon may elect to perform a simple mastectomy. Bilateral simple mastectomy is occasionally performed as a prophylactic procedure to reduce the risk of developing breast cancer. Alternatively, a patient who develops a local recurrence in the breast after breast-conserving surgery for invasive cancer may elect to undergo simple (or salvage) mastectomy. Additionally, patients with evidence of diffuse, multicentric, ductal carcinoma in situ of the breast may elect to undergo simple mastectomy.

An elliptical incision is made, incorporating the nipple–areola complex, as illustrated in Fig. 6.2. There is no need to incorporate a large amount of skin in the incision. As little skin as possible should be incorporated, as this will facilitate breast reconstruction.

The incision is taken down to the full thickness of the skin, just beyond the subcutaneous tissue. The surgical assistant then lifts up the skin edges with skin hooks or rake retractors, and the surgeon applies counter-traction on the breast with one hand and uses the other hand to dissect the breast away from the overlying subcutaneous tissue. We prefer to use a knife for this dissection, although many surgeons use electrocautery. The dissection should continue superiorly to the level of the clavicle, inferiorly to the rectus sheath, medially to the sternum, and laterally to the latissimus dorsi muscle. The breast is dissected off the pectoralis major muscle using electrocautery. The fascia overlying the pectoralis major muscle is kept intact. Throughout the dissection, meticulous attention should be paid to hemostasis.

In circumstances where the patient does not undergo immediate breast reconstruction following simple mastectomy, a Jackson–Pratt drain is brought out through a separate stab incision and the wound is closed. We generally re-approximate the subcutaneous tissue with interrupted 3–0 Vicryl, and use a running 3–0 Monocryl subcuticular stitch to re-approximate the skin edges. The Jackson–Pratt drain is attached to the skin with a 3–0 nylon stitch, and hooked to bulb suction. Dressings are applied over the wound.

6.3 Breast-Conserving Cancer Surgery

As discussed previously, if breast-conserving surgery is used to treat the cancer, then two separate incisions are generally required: one to remove the primary breast tumor and the other for the axillary dissection. The primary tumor of the breast is first extirpated, and a variety of techniques can be used, as described in the accompanying illustrations. As mentioned previously in this text, there are several terms that refer to excision of the primary tumor in breast-conserving surgery: quadrantectomy, segmental excision, and lumpectomy. Once the primary tumor is removed, the specimen is inspected to make sure that there is no evidence of gross tumor at the margins. The specimen is then oriented and the various margins (anterior, posterior, lateral, medial, superior, and inferior) are appropriately labeled using either stitches or colored ink (Fig. 5.6). The specimen is submitted to the pathologist, who determines if there is any histological evidence of tumor at the margins. If this proves to be the case, the surgeon may elect to excise additional breast tissue. Once the primary breast tumor is removed, meticulous attention is paid to hemostasis, which is achieved using electrocautery. The skin edges of the breast wound are re-approximated using a running subcuticular Monocryl stitch (3–0 or 4–0). We do not place a drain in the breast wound. A seroma generally forms in the wound, but the fluid reabsorbs over a period of several days or weeks.

The accompanying illustrations demonstrate the various techniques for local excision of breast tumors. It should be emphasized that, in most cases, an incision can be made directly over the tumor. We do not recommend "tunneling" to resect breast tumors. That is, an incision should never be made in one area of the breast requiring dissection through healthy breast tissue to extirpate a tumor in another part of the breast. We generally place an elliptical incision over the tumor, and incorporate the overlying skin with the resected specimen, particularly if the tumor is superficial. However, there are other specific techniques that can be used to extirpate primary breast tumors, and these provide good cosmetic results, as illustrated in the accompanying pages.

If the breast tumor is located centrally (immediately beneath the nipple–areola complex), then an incision is generally made incorporating the entire nipple–areola complex. The surrounding tissue is

6

undermined to obtain a clear margin around the tumor (Fig. 6.7a–d). The wound is closed with horizontal approximation of the tissue edges (Fig. 6.7a–c), or, alternatively, with an approximation that creates a small, circular and centrally located scar (Fig. 6.7d).

For tumors located beneath the nipple–areola complex, there is yet another technique that can be applied to extirpate them, particularly if their location is deep. Just below the site of resection, a skin paddle is dissected free, and tissue adjacent to it is de-epithelialized. The entire nipple–areola complex, including the tumor, is then resected down to the level of the pectoralis major muscle. The skin paddle is then advanced to fill the defect created by the tumor resection, and the skin edges re-approximated with absorbable stitches.

If the tumor is adjacent to the nipple–areola complex but not immediately beneath it, then an area around the nipple-areola complex can be de-epithelialized. The tumor is identified and extirpated, obtaining a clear margin of normal tissue around it. The dermis is then closed, and the skin re-attached to the nipple–areola complex with a running stitch as illustrated (Fig. 6.8a–g).

A similar technique can be applied for tumors located either superolateral or superomedial to the nipple–areola complex (Fig. 6.9). Again, the tissue immediately around the areola is de-epithelialized. Manual traction is applied to retract the skin further, as illustrated (Fig. 6.9c–e), thereby providing access to the tumor. The surgeon then proceeds to excise the tumor, obtaining a healthy rim of normal tissue around it. The breast tissue is then re-approximated, and the skin is re-attached to the nipple–areola complex with an absorbable stitch (Fig. 6.9f).

Resection of tumors near the nipple–areola complex may result in the retraction of the nipple–areola complex away from its central position in the breast. The nipple–areola complex may retract towards the direction of the tumor resection site (Fig. 6.10e). If this occurs, then the nipple–areola complex can be undermined and repositioned centrally (Fig. 6.10a–g).

If a breast tumor is resected from the inferior part of the breast (Fig. 6.10h, i), this may cause the breast to droop, with the nipple pointing in the downward direction. This defect can be corrected with resection of the breast tissue superiorly, providing a "breast lift," as illustrated (Fig. 6.11).

Tumors located posterior to the nipple–areola complex and extending inferiorly can be resected with a quadrantectomy, with resection of the inferior quadrant of the breast. The defect in the breast can be closed with an advancement flap taken from the upper chest wall, just below the inframammary fold. In this technique, the skin, subcutaneous tissue and fat are advanced to cover the defect in the breast, as illustrated (Fig. 6.12a–e). Posteriorly, the advancement flap is attached to the breast defect with absorbable suture, and the skin edges are also approximated with an absorbable stitch (Fig. 6.12e). The "Grisotti"-quadranectomy technique is shown in Fig. 6.12f–h.

Tumors superior or inferior to the nipple–areola complex can also be resected using the reduction mammoplasty technique described later, in Sect. 7.13. For tumors located superior to the nipple–areola complex, an incision is made around the tumor, with one arm of the incision extending medially and the other extending laterally along the nipple–areola complex, as shown in (Fig. 6.13a). The tumor is resected, and the skin edges are approximated with an absorbable stitch (Fig. 6.13b). For tumors located inferior to the nipple–areola complex, a "figure of eight" area around the nipple–areola complex and tumor is de-epithelialized, as shown (Fig. 6.13c). The tumor is then resected, and skin edges are approximated with an absorbable stitch (Fig. 6.13d).

If, following quadrantectomy, a large defect is created, this can be repaired using a prosthesis. The prosthesis should be placed below the pectoralis major muscle, as shown in Fig. 6.14.

For patients with large or locally advanced tumors, total mastectomy is not necessarily required, and breast-conserving surgery is generally possible following preoperative systemic therapy (PST). Tumor regression rates of about 80% are evident following PST, making breast-conserving surgery feasible. Prior to PST, the presence of malignant disease should be confirmed with a core biopsy, using a 14-gauge needle (or larger) to obtain at least three samples from various areas of the primary tumor.

A proposal for identifying a palpable mass before and after the clinical response to preoperative chemotherapy is shown in Fig. 6.15 [1]. Measurements are taken prior to chemotherapy to document the position of the tumor.

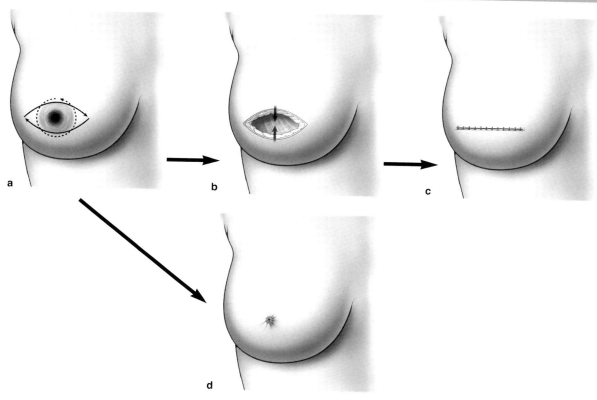

Fig. 6.7a–d. Central tumorectomy, resection of the nipple areola. a–c Wound closure with horizontal approximation of the tissue edges. a, d Wound closure creates a small, circular and centrally located scar

6

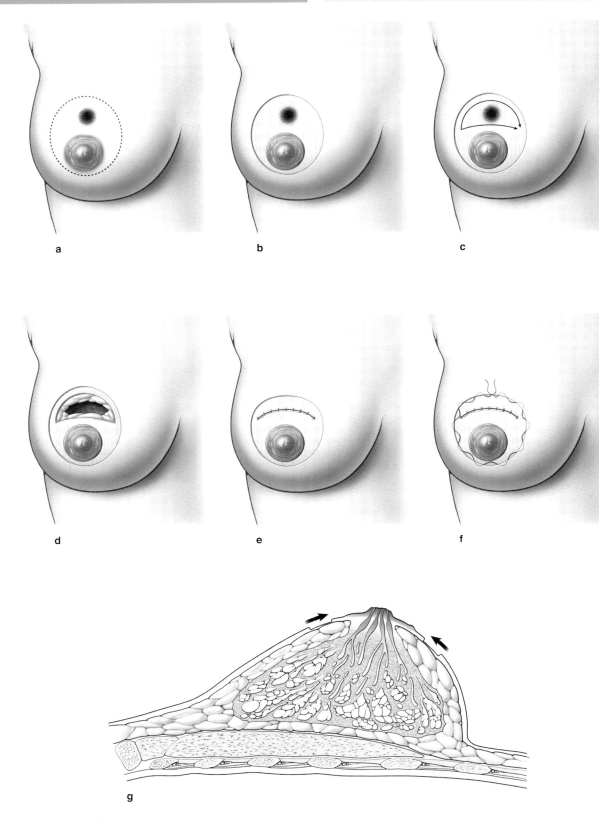

Fig. 6.8a–g. Quadrantectomy

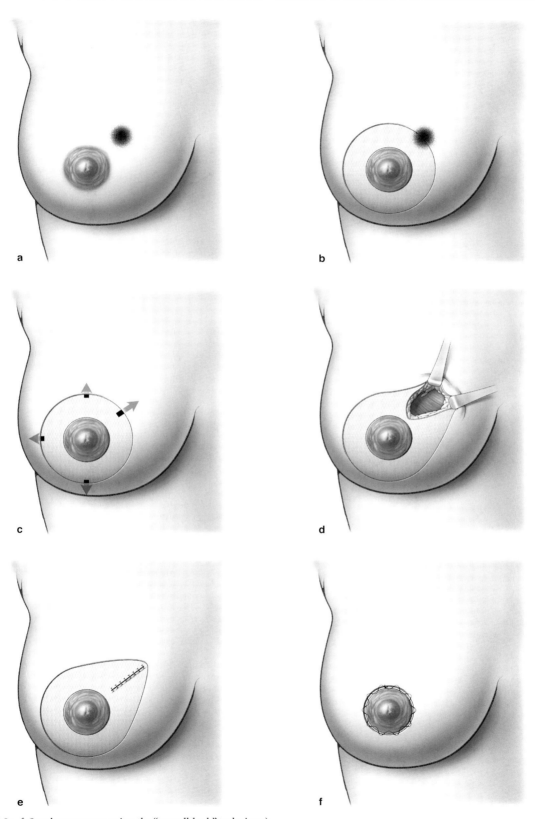

Fig. 6.9a–f. Quadrantectomy using the "roundblock" technique)

6

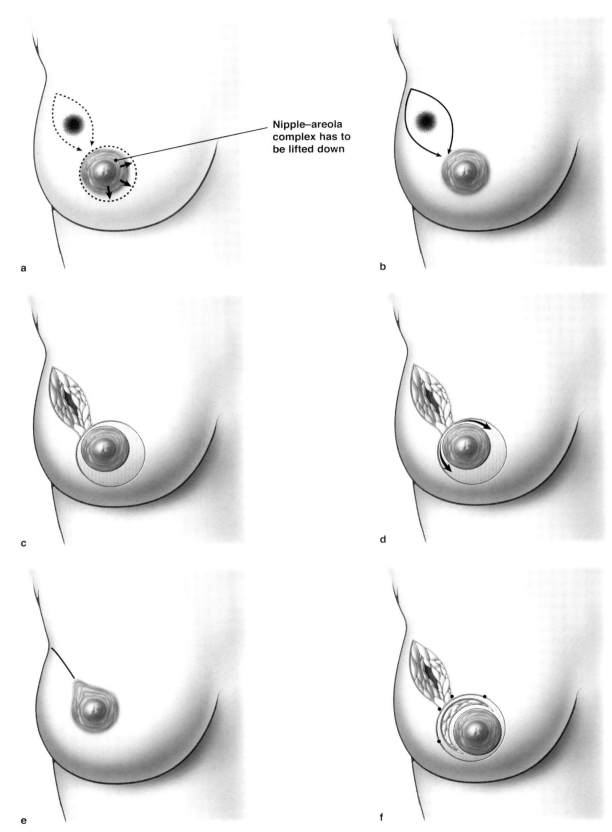

Nipple–areola
complex has to
be lifted down

a

b

c

d

e

f

Fig. 6.10a–i. Quadrantectomy

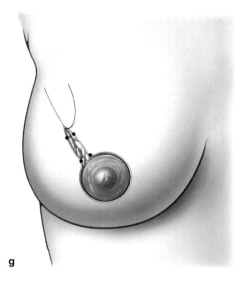

g

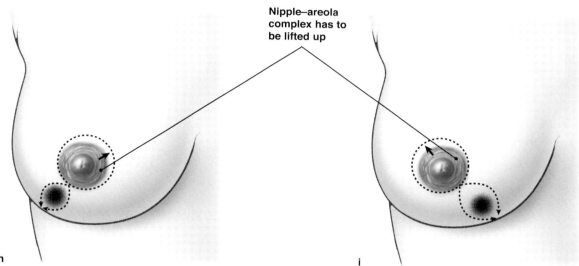

Nipple–areola complex has to be lifted up

h   i

Fig. 6.10a–i. Continued

6

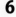
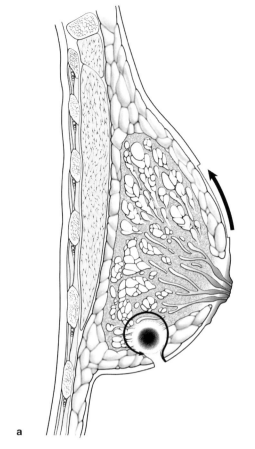
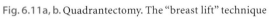
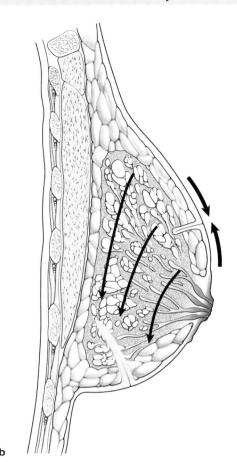

a

b

Fig. 6.11a, b. Quadrantectomy. The "breast lift" technique

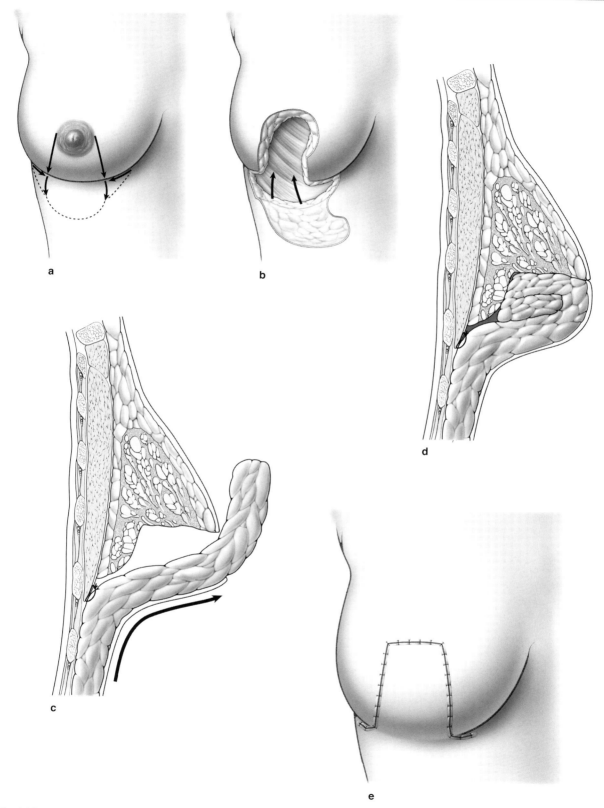

Fig. 6.12a–e. Quadrantectomy. The advancement flap/upper chest wall technique

6

Tumor underneath nipple–areola complex

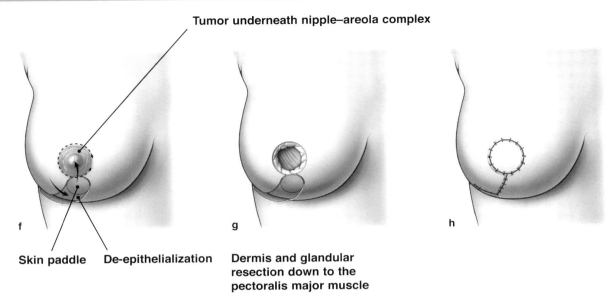

f   g   h

Skin paddle **De-epithelialization**   **Dermis and glandular
                                              resection down to the
                                              pectoralis major muscle**

Fig. 6.12f–h. Quadrantectomy "Grisotti technique"

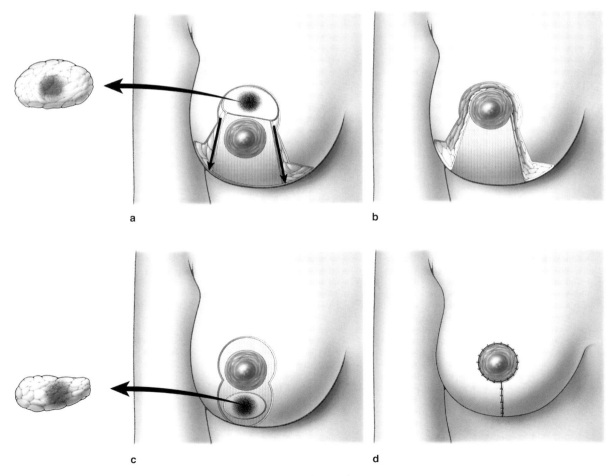

a   b

c   d

Fig. 6.13a–d. Quadrantectomy. See also the reduction mammoplasty technique

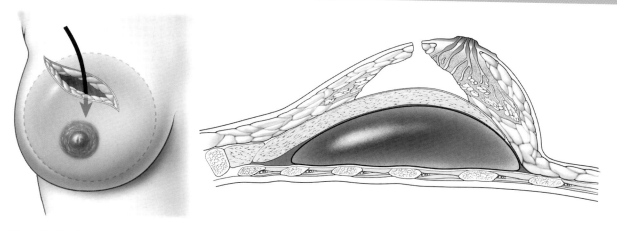

Fig. 6.14. Quadrantectomy. Partial reconstruction in the upper outer quadrant; plasty with prosthesis

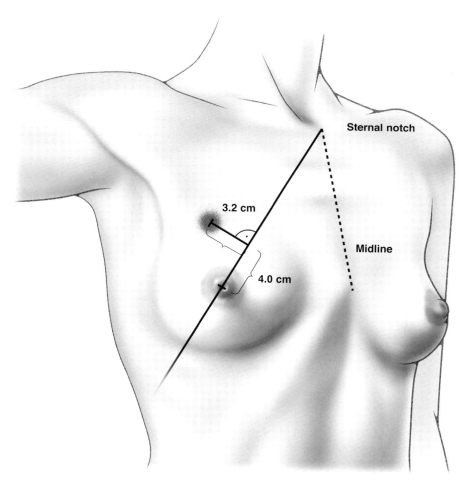

Fig. 6.15. Proposal for identifying a palpable mass before and after a clinical response to preoperative (neoadjuvant) chemo-therapy according to [1]

6.4 Axillary Lymph Node Dissection (Level I, Level II, Level III)

Figure 6.16 illustrates the relationship of the pectoralis minor muscle to the three levels of axillary dissection: level I, level II, and level III. The importance of adequately exposing the pectoralis minor muscle early in the axillary dissection should be emphasized. The axillary tissue is posterior to the pectoralis minor muscle. As shown in Fig. 6.16 a level I axillary dissection refers to extirpation of tissue lateral to the lateral border of the pectoralis minor muscle, a level II dissection refers to the removal of tissue between the medial and lateral borders of the muscle, and a level III dissection indicates tissue dissection medial to the muscle's medial border. Most surgeons generally perform only levels I and II dissection. To perform a level III dissection, the surgeon must generally divide the pectoralis minor muscle. Otherwise, it is difficult to adequately expose axillary tissue medial to the muscle.

Most surgeons generally dissect levels I and II of the axilla. If there are palpable lymph nodes lateral to the pectoralis minor muscle, then the pectoralis minor muscle is divided and a level III dissection is performed.

Following breast-conserving surgery, the axillary dissection is performed through a separate incision. This is generally placed along a skin crease, and a curving transverse incision is preferable. The incision should be placed approximately 4–5 cm below the most superior aspect of the axilla. The incision should extend anteriorly to the lateral border of the pectoralis major muscle and posteriorly to the latissimus dorsi muscle. The full thickness of the skin and underlying subcutaneous tissue are divided, and skin hooks or rake retractors used to retract the superior and inferior aspects of the wound. However, several different incision lines can be used for the axillary dissection, and these are illustrated in Fig. 6.17.

After the incision is made, attention should first be directed to the anterior aspect of the incision. Tissues are dissected down to the lateral border of the pectoralis major muscle, which is dissected free (Fig. 6.18). Care should be taken to preserve the medial and lateral pectoral nerves. The pectoralis major muscle is then retracted medially, and the lateral border of the pectoralis minor muscle is identified and dissected free (Fig. 6.18a). This dissection should continue superiorly until the axillary vein is identified (Fig. 6.18a). There is no need to continue the dissection right onto the vein. This may injure the vein and result in unnecessary bleeding. Instead, we continue the dissection along the pectoralis minor muscle superiorly until the axillary vein is visualized, with a rim of tissue immediately inferior to the vein kept intact.

The clavipectoral fascia is then divided, and we use the index fingers to gently dissect posteriorly along the chest wall until the long thoracic nerve is identified (Fig. 6.18b). This nerve is generally palpable or sometimes visualized immediately lateral to the chest wall, running in a superior to inferior direction. The long thoracic nerve innervates the serratus anterior muscle, and if it is gently pinched with forceps, the serratus anterior muscle will twitch. Care should be taken throughout the axillary dissection to keep the long thoracic nerve out of harm's way.

The pectoralis minor muscle is retracted medially, and the axillary tissue that runs posterior to the muscle is visualized. The axillary vein should again be identified at this point, and the index finger placed under the axillary tissue, and brought up just inferior to the axillary vein. The axillary tissue identified in this manner is then divided with Ligaclips. It is important to note that the extent of the axillary dissection is determined by the relationship of the dissection to the pectoralis minor muscle. The axillary tissue is posterior to the pectoralis minor muscle.

The anatomical relationship of the pectoralis minor muscle to the axillary dissection is illustrated in Figs. 6.16.

Once the superomedial extent of the axillary dissection is completed, the latissimus dorsi muscle is then identified and dissected. Keep in mind that the thoracodorsal nerve and the accompanying artery and vein enter the muscle on its medial aspect. Therefore, we identify the latissimus dorsi muscle along its lateral aspect, to avoid injury to the nerve and vessels, and then continue the dissection anteriorly. The latissimus dorsi muscle forms the lateral border of the axilla, and it should be dissected along its lateral and anterior aspect so that the surgeon can visualize the entire axilla, superiorly to the level of the axillary vein and inferiorly to the point where the latissimus dorsi muscle abuts on the chest wall.

Attention is next directed to dissection along the medial aspect of the latissimus dorsi muscle. We generally use blunt dissection (with the index fingers) to carefully identify the thoracodorsal trunk at the point where it enters the medial aspect of the latissimus dorsi muscle. Once the thoracodorsal trunk is identified, the trunk is followed superiorly to the level of the axillary vein using careful blunt dissection, and the axillary tissue anterior to the thoracodorsal trunk is extirpated and divided with Ligaclips. The thoracodorsal trunk rests on the subscapularis muscle. The entire axillary contents should, if possible, be removed as a single specimen and submitted to the pathologist.

Thus, the axillary dissection should include tissue superiorly to the level of the axillary vein, medially to the chest wall, laterally to the latissimus dorsi muscle, inferiorly to the interdigitation of the latissimus dorsi and serratus anterior muscles, and posteriorly to the subscapularis muscle. Through a separate stab incision a number 10 flat Jackson–Pratt drain is brought out from the axilla and stitched to the skin using a 3–0

nylon. The stab incision for the drain should be placed lateral to the latissimus dorsi muscle so as not to inadvertently injure any structures within the axilla. The wound is then closed with interrupted 3–0 Vicryl placed in the subcutaneous tissues, and a running 3–0 Monocryl subcuticular stitch.

Separate dressings should be applied over the axillary and breast wounds.

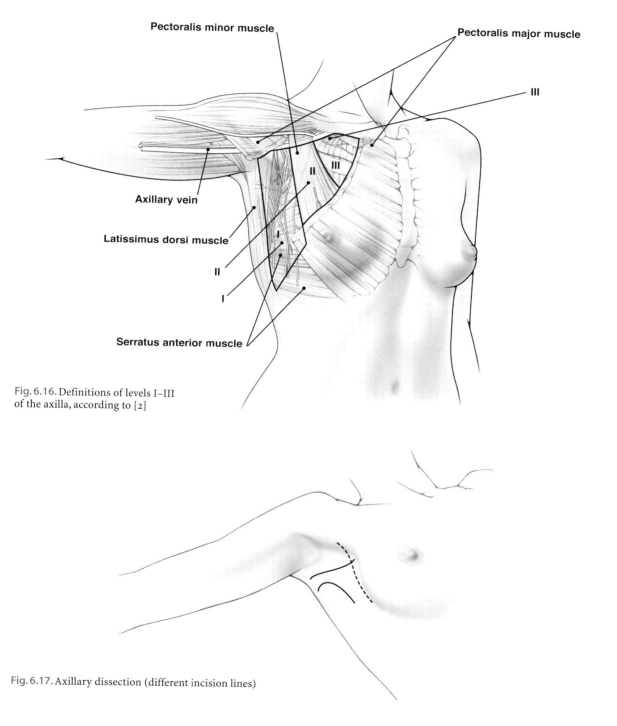

Fig. 6.16. Definitions of levels I–III of the axilla, according to [2]

Fig. 6.17. Axillary dissection (different incision lines)

6

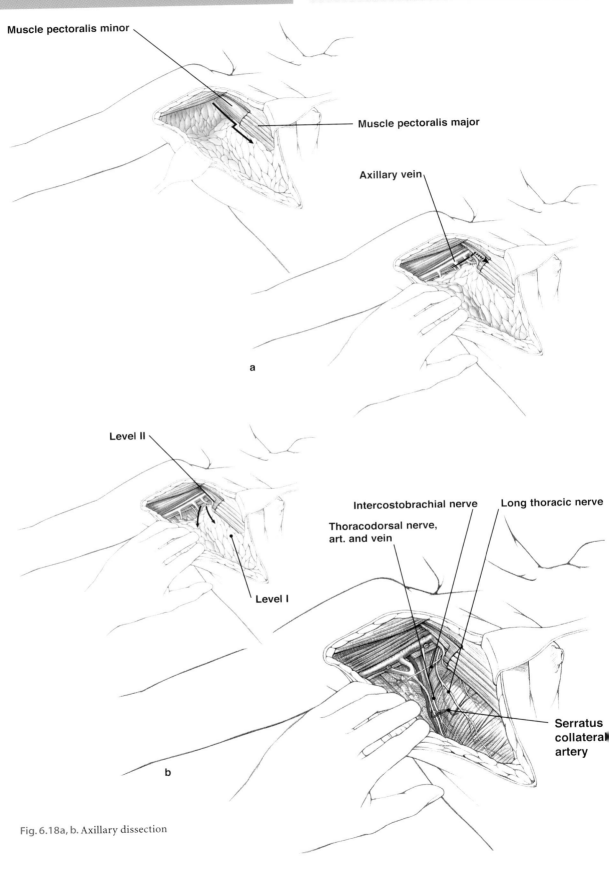

Fig. 6.18a, b. Axillary dissection

6.5 Sentinel Lymph Node Biopsy

The sentinel lymph node biopsy is a diagnostic test that is used to determine the status of the regional lymph nodes. The sentinel node is the first lymph node to receive drainage from a tumor (Fig. 6.19). It is generally assumed that if the sentinel node is free of metastatic tumor, then all other lymph nodes in the basin will also be free of tumor. Alternatively, involvement of the sentinel node indicates that other nodes in the basin may also be involved.

The surgeon identifies the sentinel lymph node by injecting blue dye and/or radioactive colloid into the breast parenchyma around the tumor or the biopsy cavity that contained the tumor (peritumoral injection) (Fig. 6.20). Some surgeons prefer to inject these lymphatic mapping agents into the plexus of lymphatics beneath the nipple–areolar complex (subareolar injection) or intradermally into the skin overlying the tumor.

There are several lymphatic mapping agents that can be used. In the United States, isosulfan blue vital dye (Lymphazurin) and/or 99m Tc sulfur colloid are generally used. In Europe, patent blue dye and/or 99m Tc albumin colloid or 99m Tc antimony trisulfide colloid are frequently used. The radiocolloid may be injected anywhere from 1 to 24 h before surgery (and the amount of colloid injected varies, depending on the projected time to surgery). However, the blue dye must be injected intraoperatively, because it passes through the sentinel lymph node after about 35 min. Thus, we generally inject 3–5 ml of the blue dye about 5 min before making the incision to identify the sentinel lymph node. The choice of lymphatic mapping agent is primarily determined by the surgeon's preference. Some surgeons use only blue dye, others use only radioactive colloid, and some use both.

The lymphatic mapping agents are carried from the breast by afferent lymphatics, and the lymph node that initially traps the dye and/or radiocolloid is identified as the sentinel lymph node. Surgeons who use only blue dye will generally make a small incision in the axillary crease, and dissect down into the axilla. The afferent lymphatic containing the blue dye is identified and followed until the bluish-colored sentinel lymph node is identified. If radiocolloid is used, then the sentinel lymph node is identified by the radioactivity counts emitted from the node and recorded by a hand-held gamma probe (Fig. 6.21). It should be noted that more than one sentinel lymph node is sometimes identified.

Once the sentinel lymph node is identified, it is dissected free and resected by applying Ligaclips or ties to the lymphatics around it and then dividing between the ligatures. The sentinel node is submitted for histological evaluation. If there is no evidence of metastatic disease in the sentinel lymph node, then most surgeons will not perform a complete axillary lymph node dissection, and the small axillary wound is closed with a running subcuticular stitch (we use either 3-0 or 4-0 Monocryl). A drain is not placed in the axilla, as is generally done for a complete axillary dissection. However, if there is evidence of metastatic disease in the sentinel lymph node, then the patient will generally undergo a completion axillary lymph node dissection, using the techniques described earlier in this text.

Sentinel lymph node biopsy is relatively new technology, and there are still many unanswered questions concerning how best to manage patients following such a biopsy. Several large randomized prospective trials have been initiated to address these questions. Thus, the overall long-term effects of omitting axillary clearance in sentinel node-negative patients have not been fully elucidated.

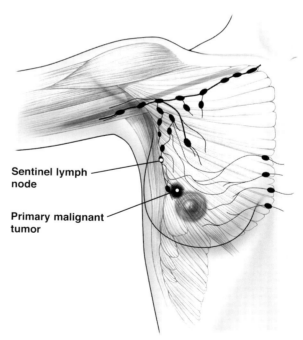

Sentinel lymph node

Primary malignant tumor

Fig. 6.19. Sentinel lymph node

6

depots of activity

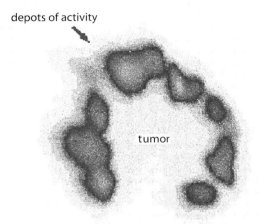

tumor

Pinhole after application

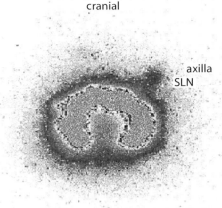

left thorax (anterior–posterior)
after 17 hours after radiocolloid application

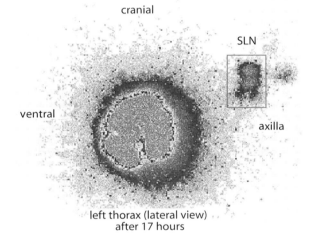

left thorax (lateral view)
after 17 hours

Fig. 6.20. Identification of sentinel lymph node (SLN). Breast cancer left side, upper outside quadrant

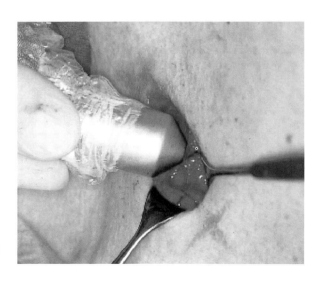

Fig. 6.21. Intraoperative sentinel lymph node detection in the axilla by hand-held gamma detector

6.6 Internal Mammary Node Biopsy

The advent of sentinel lymph node biopsy has generated considerable interest in the potential significance of metastasis to the internal mammary nodes. In patients with primary breast cancer, the internal mammary nodal chain is the most important drainage site outside the axilla. When radiocolloid is used as a lymphatic mapping agent, either alone or in conjunction with blue dye, a lymphoscintigram may be performed preoperatively to visualize the location of the sentinel lymph node. In such instances, metastasis to the internal mammary nodes has been reported in about 27% of all patients with primary breast cancer, with about 7% having metastasis to the internal mammary nodes and not to the axillary nodes.

Internal mammary sentinel node biopsy is not standard practice. We still do not know if information gathered from internal mammary node biopsy will improve outcome in patients with primary breast cancer. In our opinion, at the present time, this procedure should be considered investigational and only performed in a clinical trial setting.

The injection of radiocolloid for sentinel lymph node biopsy is described in the previous section (Sect. 6.5). A preoperative lymphoscintigram may reveal metastases to the internal mammary nodes. The surgeon may then elect to take a biopsy of the internal mammary sentinel node (generally in a clinical trial setting). Metastases to the internal mammary nodes are usually located in the first or second intercostal spaces. Intraoperatively, the surgeon identifies the site of the internal mammary sentinel node using a hand-held gamma probe (Fig. 6.22). A small incision is made overlying the intercostal space containing the internal mammary node, and tissue is dissected down to the node. The node is excised after ligating the lymphatics around it (with either 3–0 or 4–0 silk ties or Ligaclips) and then dividing these lymphatics. The internal mammary node is then removed and submitted to the pathologist for histological evaluation. Electrocautery is used to achieve hemostasis in the wound. The small skin incision is closed primarily with interrupted 3–0 or 4–0 nylon stitches, and dressings are applied over the wound.

6.7 Venous Access for Chemotherapy

Several large, randomized prospective trials have shown that adjuvant chemotherapy can reduce breast mortality. Thus, many patients will require multiple courses of intravenous chemotherapy following surgery for primary breast cancer, and the use of venous access ports facilitates administration of such therapy (Fig. 6.22). Obviously, patients who are treated only with oral endocrine agents following surgery for primary breast cancer will not require placement of venous access catheters.

There are two types of venous access catheters: those placed beneath the skin, and those placed percutaneously and covered with a sterile dressing. In each case, either single-lumen or double-lumen catheters are available.

When placing a catheter for venous access, careful attention should be paid to assure that a sterile technique is applied, so as to reduce the risk of introducing infection. The patient should be placed in the supine position, with arms at the side. A wide area around the delto-pectoral groove is cleaned with a sterilizing solution, such as Betadine®, and sterile drapes placed around the field. In most cases, local anesthesia with intravenous sedation is all that is required.

A small incision, measuring about 3–5 cm, is made in the delto-pectoral groove, and tissues are carefully dissected down until the cephalic vein is identified. The cephalic vein is dissected free to allow the placement of two ties (we use 3–0 silk), with a distance of about 2 cm between the ties. The distal tie is used to ligate the cephalic vein.

The mediport with the attached catheter should now be ready for placement. Using blunt dissection, a pocket is dissected below the skin and above the pectoralis major muscle for placement of the mediport. Next, the required length of the catheter tubing is measured by extending it from the planned insertion site to the angle of Louis. The excess catheter tubing is cut distally.

A 15-blade knife is used to make a small opening on the anterior aspect of the cephalic vein (between the two ties), and the catheter passed proximally into the axillary vein. The entire length of the catheter, as previously measured, should be passed into the vein. Once this is accomplished, the correct positioning of the catheter should be verified by fluoroscopy. The proximal ligature on the cephalic vein is then tied down to secure the catheter in place. The mediport is immobilized in its pocket by attaching it to the underlying fascia with interrupted nonabsorbable sutures. After closing the skin, the patency of the mediport should be confirmed with percutaneous placement of a syringe containing heparinized saline. Blood should be aspirated through the port and heparinized saline solution flushed through it.

Alternatively, the mediport catheter can be inserted following direct puncture of the subclavian vein. A rolled towel is generally placed between the scapulae to facilitate such a puncture. There are several kits commercially available that provide the necessary instrumentation for subclavian vein catheterization. Following subclavian puncture, the catheter tubing is generally passed over a guide wire into the vein, and the insertion site is extended and a pocket created for placement of the mediport. The mediport should be attached to the underlying fascia with interrupted nonabsorbable sutures. An alternative venous access will be the cephalic or jugular vein (Fig. 6.22).

References

1. Kaufmann M, von Minckwitz G, Smith R et al (2003) International expert panel on the use of primary (preoperative) systemic treatment of operable breast cancer: review and recommendations. J Clin Oncol 21(3):2600–2608
2. Berg JW (1955) The significance of axillary node levels in the study of breast carcinoma. Cancer 8:776–778

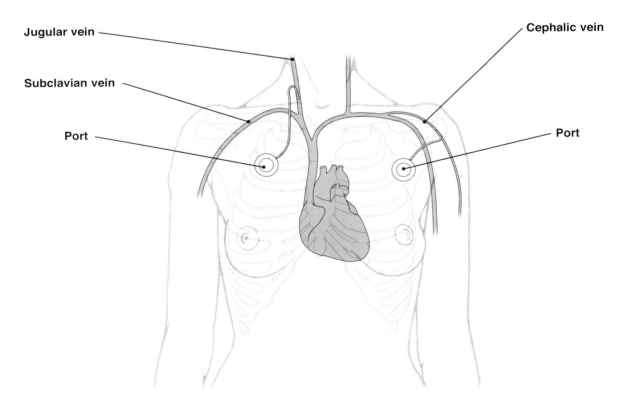

Fig. 6.22. Venous access for chemotherapy

Chapter 7

Plastic and Reconstructive Breast Surgery

7.1 Immediate and Delayed Breast Reconstruction

Following mastectomy for breast cancer, reconstructive surgery reduces anxiety and thereby improves the quality of life for many women. Breast reconstruction can be done at the time of the mastectomy (immediate breast reconstruction), or at any time after the mastectomy (delayed breast reconstruction). In recent years, immediate breast reconstruction has gained wider acceptance. Breast reconstruction can be performed using either prostheses or autogenous tissue.

There are several options available for those patients choosing prostheses. A permanent prosthesis can be placed at the time of mastectomy. Alternatively, an expander can be placed, and inflated gradually over a period of several weeks by injecting solution through a port. This results in the creation of a ptosis. The injectable port and expander are then removed and replaced with a permanent prosthesis, or, in some cases, the expander is left in place as the permanent prosthesis.

For those patients choosing reconstruction with autogenous tissue, the two most widely accepted options are the latissimus dorsi flap and the transverse rectus abdominis muscle (TRAM) flap. The latissimus dorsi muscle flap does not provide sufficient tissue bulk, and a prosthesis is generally placed beneath the flap. However, a new technique promoted by Delay [1] in France provides satisfactory results in selected patients, using the latissimus dorsi flap without placement of an implant.

In contrast, the TRAM flap provides considerable tissue bulk, and, in most cases, a prosthesis is not required. The TRAM flap is technically a much more difficult surgical procedure, and carries with it a greater risk of complications. A large number of different TRAM flap techniques have been developed, including pedicled and free flaps that require the use of microvascular procedures. The aim of the free flaps is to minimize the amount of muscle removed from the abdominal wall.

7.2 Placement of Definitive Prosthesis

The accompanying illustrations depict the technique of immediate breast reconstruction following a Patey mastectomy (modified radical mastectomy; Fig. 6.1), with placement of a definitive prosthesis. Prior to surgery, the surgeon should assess the amount of redundant abdominal wall tissue (Fig. 7.1a). This is necessary because this tissue will have to be mobilized superiorly for placement of a prosthesis, and a new inframammary fold will need to be created. Also, following mastectomy, the lateral border of the removed breast should be marked on the muscles, to avoid placing part of the prosthesis in the axilla.

After mastectomy, curved scissors and blunt dissection are used to create a space between the pectoralis major and pectoralis minor muscles. A plane between these muscles is identified laterally, and a large area within that plane is dissected free (Fig. 7.1b). Also, extending inferiorly, the skin and subcutaneous tissue anterior to the rectus abdominis muscle should now be mobilized and dissected free (see Fig. 6.6.1a–c). The mobilization of this tissue is necessary because, once the prosthesis is placed under the pectoralis major muscle, additional skin and subcutaneous tissue will be required to close the wound over the pectoralis major muscle (see Fig. 6.6.1d–f).

The superolateral border of the pectoralis major muscle is dissected free and undermined, leaving the pectoralis minor muscle intact. The lateral extent of the dissection continues beneath the serratus anterior muscle, and should stop at the predetermined lateral border of the breast (Fig. 7.2, 7.3). The undermining of the pectoralis major muscle then continues with blunt and sharp dissection medially to the level of the sternum (Fig. 7.4). This dissection continues medially on the sternum as far as necessary to duplicate the opposite breast. The limits of the medial aspect of the pectoral undermining are illustrated. Undermining of the pectoralis major muscle continues with detachment of its insertions as shown, according to the levels a, b, and c. Then 3–0 Vicryl sutures are placed at the muscle openings and left untied. Once the prosthesis or expander is fitted into the muscular pocket, the sutures are tied down. Also, dissection of the muscular pocket should continue to the inferior extent of the pectoralis major muscle.

As illustrated, immediate breast reconstruction following mastectomy can be achieved with placement of a definitive prosthesis within the muscular pocket (Fig. 7.5a). This pocket is comprised of the pectoralis and serratus anterior muscles. Once the prosthesis is placed in the muscular pocket, the pock-

et should be closed with absorbable stitches. However, if the pectoralis muscle is wide enough, and if the lateral aspect of the skin is well supplied with blood, the muscular pocket can be left open laterally after placement of the prosthesis. Two Jackson–Pratt drains are generally left in the muscular pocket and brought out laterally after closure of the wound (Fig. 7.5b). These drains are hooked to bulb suction, and removed postoperatively once drainage is minimal (about 30 ml/day from each drain).

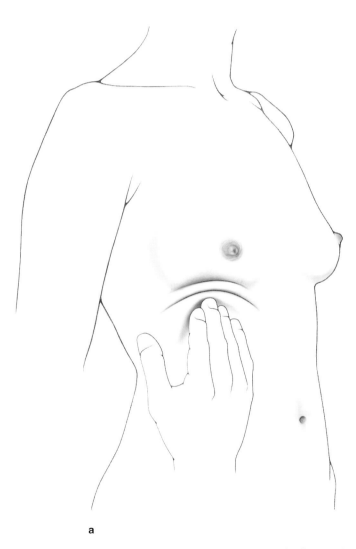

a

Fig. 7.1a, b. Immediate breast reconstruction using the "suspension technique". A new mammary fold is created to bring tissue up before putting in a prosthesis

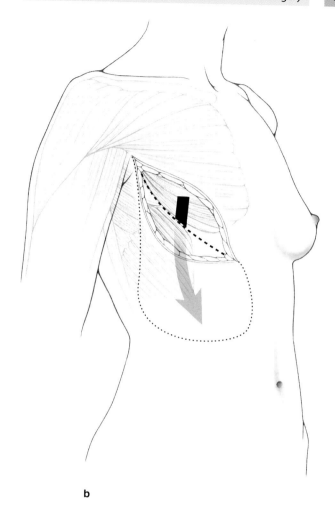

b

Fig. 7.1a, b. Immediate breast reconstruction using the "suspen-sion technique". A new mammary fold is created to bring tissue up before putting in a prosthesis

7

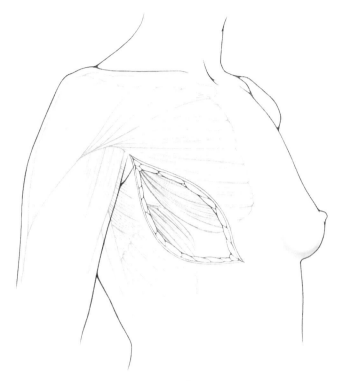

Fig. 7.2. Immediate reconstruction after Patey mastectomy

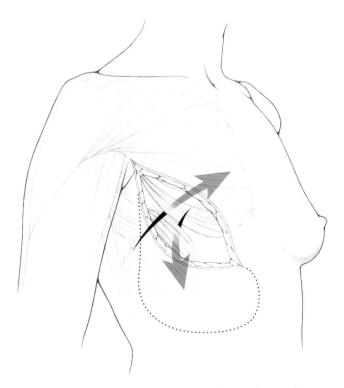

Fig. 7.3. Serratus muscle is brought up and pectoralis muscle brought down to create a pocket for a prosthesis

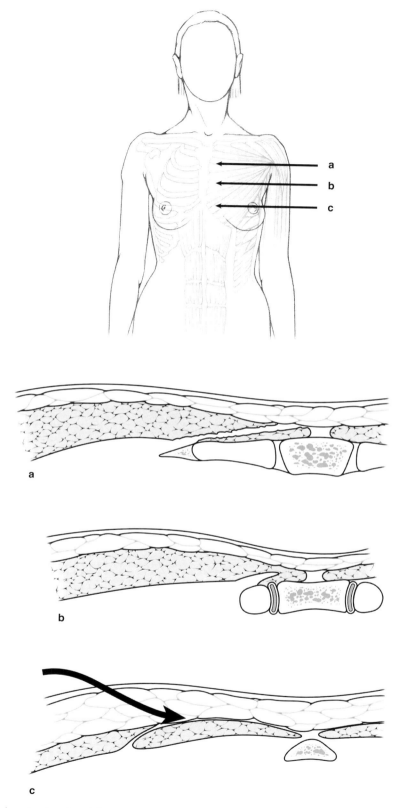

Fig. 7.4. Limits of the subpectoral undermining

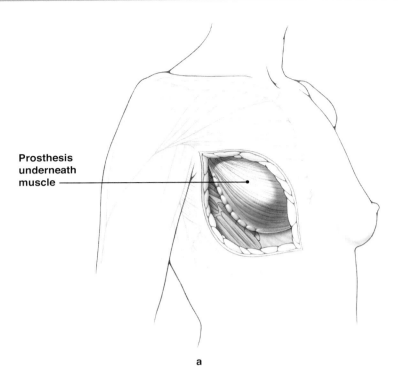

Prosthesis
underneath
muscle

a

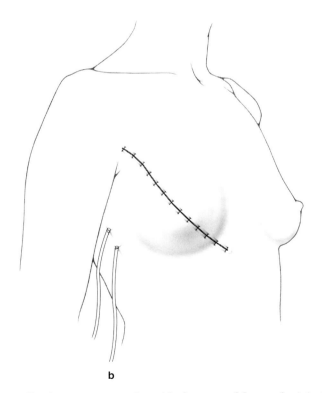

b

Fig. 7.5a, b. Immediate breast reconstruction, with placement of the prosthesis in the muscular pocket

7.3 Breast Reconstruction with Expander

A muscular pocket is created, as described previously for placement of a definitive prosthesis. The pocket is comprised of the pectoralis major and serratus anterior muscles. The expander is placed in the muscular pocket and the catheter and port are tunneled and brought to a position under the skin in the axilla (Fig. 7.6).

Alternatively, in some cases, the port is located on the surface of the implant itself (Fig. 7.7). When the port is located on the sheet of the implant itself, a magnetic device can help to localize the port and thereby guide the inflation.

The expander is inflated by passing a 22-gauge needle through the port and injecting saline solution through it. This is done once or twice each week until the expander is inflated such that the area of the nipple projection is at the same level bilaterally. This will provide a degree of ptosis. After suitable expansion, the expander is replaced by a permanent prosthesis.

Figures 7.6 and 7.7a, b illustrate the principle of cutaneous expansion, which is necessary to obtain a degree of ptosis. The ptosis is achieved with gradual inflation of the prosthesis by injecting saline solution through the port once or twice each week over a period of several weeks. An over-expansion is recommended by many surgeons, in order to gain the additional tissue required for a more natural ptosis.

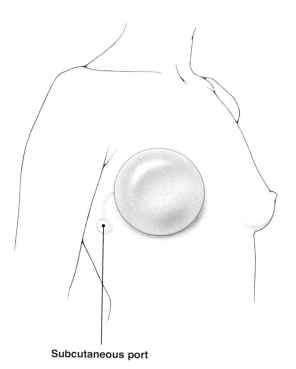

Subcutaneous port

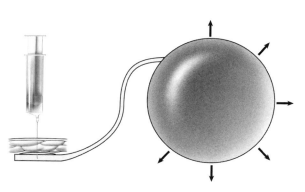

Fig. 7.6. Breast reconstruction with expander

7

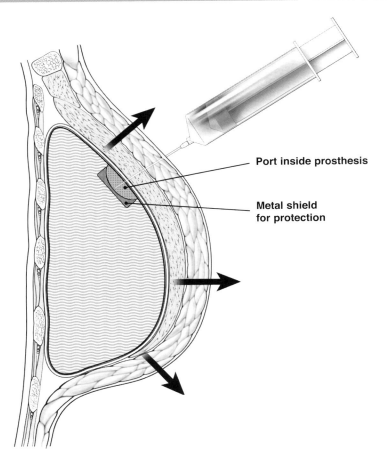

Port inside prosthesis

Metal shield
for protection

Fig. 7.7a. Cutaneous expander

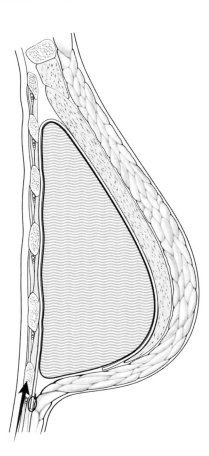

Fig. 7.7b. Position of the definitive prosthesis. After definitive substitution with a definitive prothesis same stiches in the sulcus improve the natural ptosis

7.4 Hypothesis to Explain Capsular Contracture

Specialized fibroblasts that have the ability to contract will migrate to the area around breast implants and expanders. These contractile fibroblasts, known as myofibroblasts, are responsible for wound contraction, and seem also to be responsible for capsular contraction. After a wound heals, myofibroblasts generally disappear. However, myofibroblasts persist in capsules that form around breast prostheses, and this might explain the mechanism for capsular contracture [2].

As shown in the accompanying illustrations, when an implant is placed in the breast, it becomes lined with contractile fibroblasts (Fig. 7.8). Thus, the implant can be viewed as a three-dimensional wound. The contractile fibroblasts are responsible for initial contracture, but pressure from the implant prevents further contracture. Firmer implants should therefore be less prone to capsular contracture than softer implants. If the implant ruptures, this may result in a worse contracture.

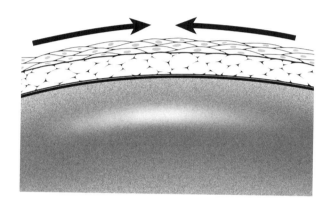

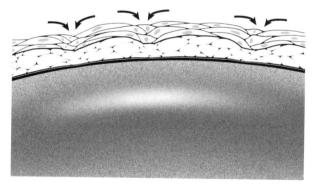

Fig. 7.8. A hypothesis to explain capsular contracture

7.5 Suspension Technique (Advancement Abdominal Flap)

If a permanent prosthesis is to be placed following a mastectomy, the cosmetic appearance can often be improved with the "suspension technique." First, a wide area of abdominal tissue is undermined inferiorly, just along the anterior surface of the rectus abdominis muscle (Fig. 7.9a). In this manner, the skin and subcutaneous tissue along the inferior aspect of the mastectomy wound are mobilized. The head of the operating table should then be raised, placing the patient in a semi-sitting position. The abdominal flap that has been mobilized is then pulled up and maintained with a triangular nonabsorbable mesh that is fixed at the level of the future inframammary fold. The mesh is brought up superiorly, posterior to the pectoralis major muscle, as shown (Figs. 7.9b, 7.10), and the superior aspect of the mesh is attached to the costal cartilage with two nonabsorbable stitches (3–0 Prolene), as depicted in the illustration (Fig. 7.9b). The prosthesis is placed anterior to the mesh and posterior to the pectoralis muscle as shown (Fig. 7.10). This "suspension technique," or abdominal flap advancement, was first described by Rietjens [3].

7

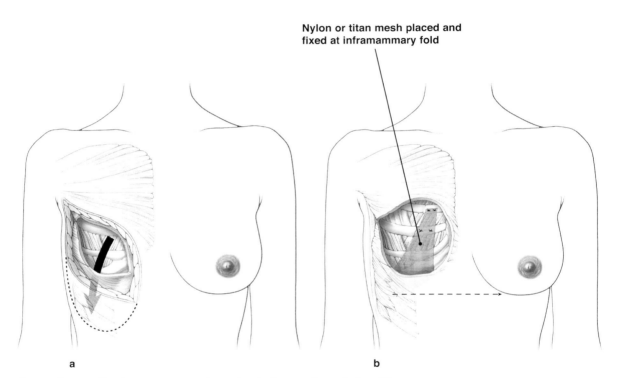

Nylon or titan mesh placed and fixed at inframammary fold

a   b

Fig. 7.9a, b. Immediate breast reconstruction, using the "suspension technique II"

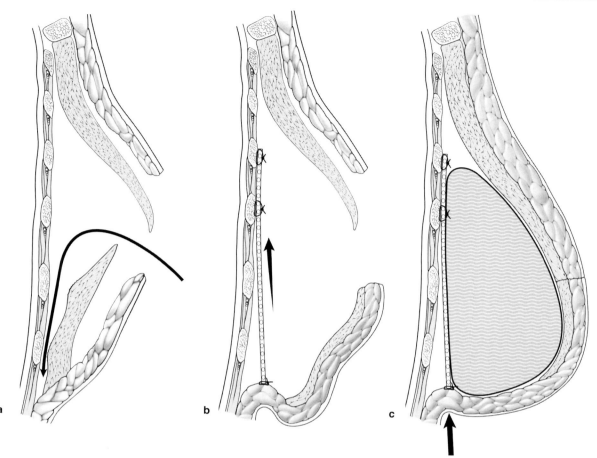

a

b

c

Fig. 7.10. a Immediate breast reconstruction using the "suspension technique" (profile view). b With mesh. c Suspension technique with mesh and subpectoral prothesis

7.6 Latissimus Dorsi Flap

Prior to surgery, the surgeon should outline the site of the planned mastectomy skin incision with indelible ink. This same incision pattern is outlined on paper, which is then used as a template to outline the skin over the latissimus dorsi muscle (Fig. 7.11). The accompanying illustration depicts the possible different locations of the skin paddles overlying the latissimus dorsi muscle that might be used in a latissimus dorsi flap (Fig. 7.11). The more elliptical the skin incision, the generally easier it is to close.

The latissimus dorsi flap is comprised of the skin paddle and underlying fat and muscle (Fig. 7.12).

When the latissimus dorsi flap is used for immediate breast reconstruction, the mastectomy must be completed before beginning the reconstruction. The mastectomy wound is packed with moist laparotomy pads, and isolated with a vinyl drape. The patient is then turned on her side and placed in the lateral decubitus position, providing the surgeon with easy access to the latissimus dorsi muscle and surrounding tissues. The patient's position on the operating room table is secured with a bean bag.

An elliptical incision is made on the previously marked surface of the skin overlying the latissimus dorsi muscle. The incision is taken down to the muscle, and an area of adjacent skin is undermined. The latissimus dorsi flap is mobilized, incising muscle along its anterior margin and continuing the dissection posteriorly, using fingers to bluntly dissect the muscle off the underlying rib cage. When the posterior attachments of the flap are freed, its peripheral attachments are severed by sharp dissection, beginning inferiorly and continuing the dissection superiorly. Along the superior aspect of the dissection, care should be taken to identify and preserve the thoracodorsal pedicle, which should have been previously exposed during the axillary dissection. Preservation of the thoracodorsal pedicle is critical, as it provides the blood supply to the latissimus dorsi flap. With blunt dissection, a tunnel is created from the mastectomy defect into the axilla, and the tunnel enlarged sufficiently to allow the pedicle of the latissimus dorsi flap to be rotated into the mastectomy defect.

The back wound (from which the latissimus dorsi flap was taken) is closed primarily, with a Jackson–Pratt drain brought out inferior to the wound. The wound is generally closed in two layers, with interrupted 3–0 Vicryl sutures for the deep dermal layer, followed by a running 3–0 subcuticular Monocryl stitch placed superficially. Once the back wound is closed, the bean bag is deflated and removed, and the patient is again rotated to the supine position to complete the reconstruction on the anterior chest wall. The vinyl drape overlying the mastectomy wound is removed, the patient is re-prepped and re-draped, and the surgeon is now ready to secure the flap onto the anterior chest wall.

The pectoralis major muscle is detached from its origin on the ribs and sutured to the superior aspect of the latissimus dorsi muscle. The inferior aspect of the latissimus dorsi muscle is sutured into the rectus abdominis muscle, and the lateral aspect of the latissimus dorsi is sutured to the serratus anterior muscle. In this manner, a submuscular pocket is created. A few of these sutures are left untied, and prostheses of various sizes are placed into this pocket, until one of suitable size is found. The appropriately-sized prosthesis is left in place, and the sutures are tied down around it. Skin edges of the wound are then re-approximated (Fig. 7.12).

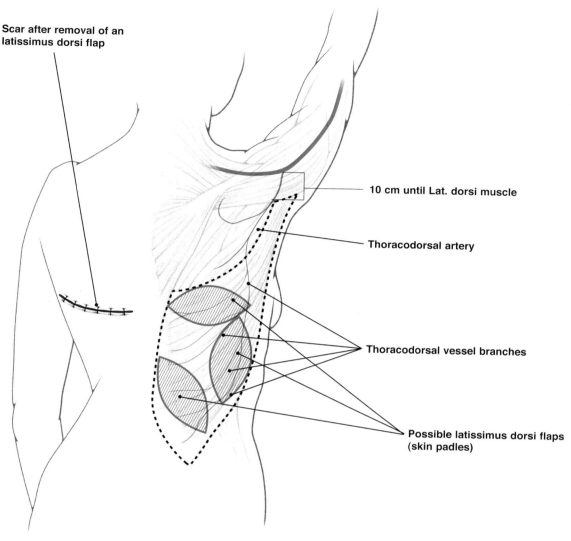

Scar after removal of an latissimus dorsi flap

10 cm until Lat. dorsi muscle

Thoracodorsal artery

Thoracodorsal vessel branches

Possible latissimus dorsi flaps (skin padles)

Fig. 7.11. Breast reconstruction with latissimus dorsi flap, blood supply and possible skin padles

7

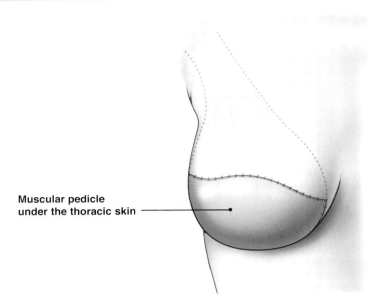

Muscular pedicle
under the thoracic skin

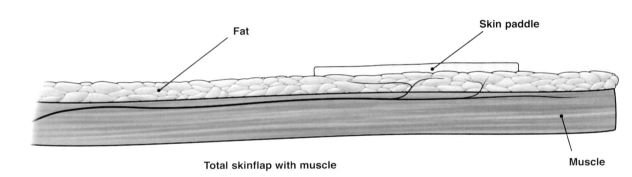

Fat

Skin paddle

Total skinflap with muscle

Muscle

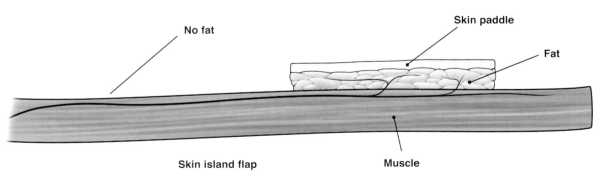

No fat

Skin paddle

Fat

Skin island flap

Muscle

Fig. 7.12. Latissimus dorsi flap

7.7 Total Breast Reconstruction with a Totally De-epithelialized Latissimus Dorsi Flap and Autologous Latissimus Flap

The accompanying illustration depicts breast reconstruction with a totally de-epithelialized latissimus dorsi flap (Fig. 7.13).

The latissimus dorsi flap (with its de-epithelialized skin paddle) is mobilized and brought into the mastectomy wound as previously described. The de-epithelialized skin paddle is buried under the thoracic skin and folded on itself. The skin from the anterior surface of the chest wall is then re-approximated, with the latissimus dorsi flap and its de-epithelialized skin paddle buried underneath. This flap provides a mound of tissue beneath the thoracic skin, simulating the breast. Such a procedure, especially when performed according to the method described by Delay [1] in France, provides enough tissue bulk to create a breast mound without the need for a prosthesis. Bulk is increased thanks to the extensive harvesting of the muscle covered by subcutaneous fat, resulting in a fatty flap vascularized by the margins of the muscle. New procedures offer preparation of the de-epithelialized latissimus flap by endoscopic preparation.

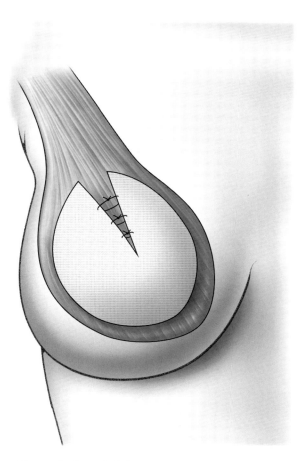

Fig. 7.13. Total breast reconstruction with a totally de-epithelialized latissimus dorsi flap. The de-epithelialized skin paddle is buried under the thoracic skin and folded on itself

7.8 Latissimus Dorsi Flap to Repair Glandular Defects Following Quadrantectomy

Following breast-conserving surgery, a large glandular defect in the upper outer quadrant can be repaired with a latissimus dorsi flap tunneled into the wound, as depicted in these illustrations. The tissue bulk provided by the latissimus flap improves the cosmetic outcome following breast-conserving surgery (Fig. 7.14a–c).

7

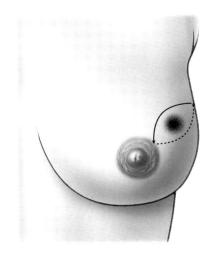

a

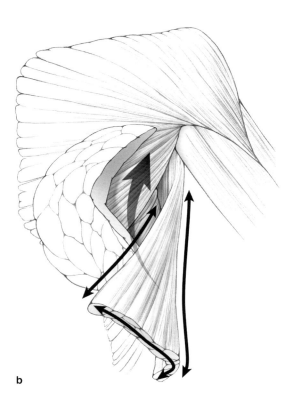

b

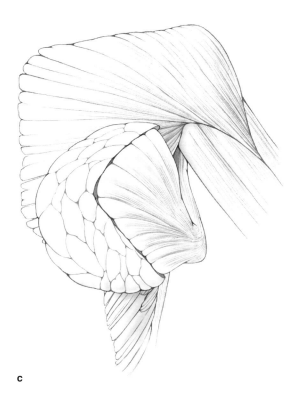

c

Fig. 7.15a–c. Quadrantectomy. Glandular defect in the upper outer quadrant; plasty with muscular latissimus dorsi flap

7.9 Pedicle TRAM Flap Reconstruction

Prior to surgery, with the patient standing, the breast is outlined with indelible ink. The perimeter of the flap to be taken from the abdominal wall is also outlined. This is done by grasping tissue approximately two finger breadths above and below the umbilicus and pulling up on the anterior abdominal wall as much as possible with two hands. The surgeon should make certain, by gently pinching the superior and inferior aspects of this tissue, that the edges will easily re-approximate once the flap is taken, and the patient is in a sitting position (Fig. 7.15).

The key anatomical structure within the TRAM flap, is, of course, the rectus abdominis muscle. The rectus abdominis is situated within longitudinal fascial sheaths on the anterior abdominal wall, and is readily visible once the skin and subcutaneous tissues of the anterior abdominal wall are retracted anteriorly. The blood supply of the rectus abdominis is derived from the superior epigastric artery (a contin-

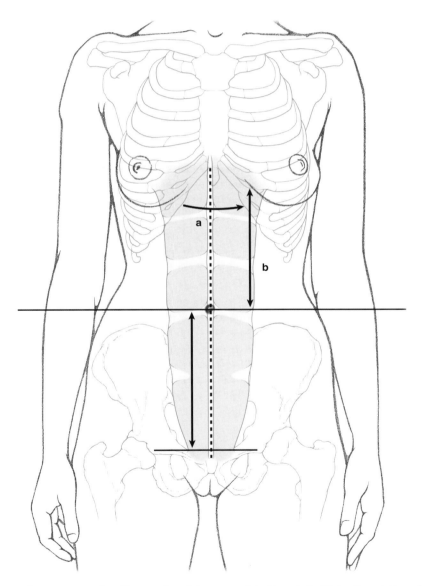

Fig. 7.15. Pedicle TRAM flap reconstruction. The opening of the costo–xiphoid angle facilitates the rotation of the superior portion of the pedicle (*a*). The distance between the umbilicus and the costal border corresponds to the real length of the pedicle and helps to predict whether the pedicle will be tense or not after transfer of the flap (*b*)

uation of the internal mammary artery) and the inferior epigastric artery (from the external iliac artery). These vessels enter the posterior aspect of the rectus abdominis muscles. Additional blood supply is derived from the intercostal vessels, which enter the rectus abdominis muscles laterally. The blood supply to the overlying skin is largely derived from perforating branches of the underlying muscles. Thus, branches of the epigastric vessels perforate through the anterior rectus sheath and supply the skin.

The skin on the abdominal wall, as previously outlined, is incised, sharply cutting down to the level of the fascia. Then, skin and subcutaneous tissues are undermined superiorly up to the level of the xiphoid. During this dissection, a plane is developed between the subcutaneous tissues and underlying muscle fascia.

The portion of the flap (the random portion) that will not be attached to the underlying rectus muscle is elevated off the contralateral rectus fascia and brought to the midline (the medial aspect of the rectus sheath) (Fig. 7.16).

It is generally recommended that the random portion of the flap paddle is left attached to the rectus until harvesting of the main pedicle is completed. Therefore, in the event that the superior epigastric vessels of the main pedicle are injured, there is still the option of using the contralateral pedicle.

Thus, the random portion is composed of skin and subcutaneous tissue, with no underlying muscle. Additionally, the ipsilateral random portion is dissected off the external oblique fascia and brought to the lateral aspect of the rectus sheath. The skin overlying the rectus muscle (which will be included in the TRAM flap) is supplied with a row of medial and lateral perforating vessels. Care should be taken to preserve these vessels.

At this point, the surgeon divides the inferior rectus fascia (below the TRAM flap), and identifies the muscle. The surgeon places two fingers underneath the rectus muscle and lifts it anteriorly, thereby placing it under tension. The inferior epigastric pedicle should now be palpable. The muscle is then divided, and the inferior epigastric pedicle is doubly ligated with 3-0 silk and divided. The rectus muscle is dissected free posteriorly and the lateral aspect of the rectus sheath is divided with a scalpel up to the superior border of the flap. The medial border of the rectus sheath is divided to the level of the umbilicus, which is then dissected free from the flap (Fig. 7.17).

The fascia overlying the rectus muscle is then incised up to the level of the xiphoid (Fig. 7.18). The rectus muscle is completely mobilized by sharp and blunt dissection, and a tunnel created through the inframammary fold, communicating with the mastectomy wound. The flap is then rotated into the wound (Figs. 7.19, 7.20). The muscle layer of the flap is sutured to the surrounding pectoralis major muscle, and skin edges are approximated. Jackson–Pratt drains are placed in the axilla and the upper abdomen.

Closure of the abdominal wounds is depicted in the accompanying illustrations (Figs. 7.21, 7.22).

An imbricating running suture is placed in the opposite anterior rectus sheath to help bring the umbilicus to the midline and thereby provide symmetry (Fig. 7.23a–c). In most cases of bipedicle flap reconstruction, a mesh closure is generally necessary (Fig. 7.21a–c).

7.9.1 Abdominal Closure

The closure of the abdomen is a major step of the operation, and should be done meticulously to avoid complications such as skin necrosis, hernia, and unsightly scars. The suture of the fascia should be done with the patient in the lying position while the closure of the cutaneous flaps will be done at the end in a sitting position.

The fascia can be closed directly with nonabsorbable stitches under moderate tension and without mesh in the case of a single pedicle. When the fascia seems fragile and when the tension is important we recommend inserting a mesh (Fig. 7.22). A nonabsorbable mesh is more secure and can be totally covered by the superficial layer of the rectus fascia. In the case of a double pedicle, mesh is required to prevent further herniation. Closure of the fascia in a single pedicle creates strong tension on the umbilicus that does not remain on the median line of the abdomen.

Centralization of the umbilicus can be obtained thanks to a plicature of the fascia of the opposite muscle as shown in Fig. 7.23a–c.

It is also possible to create the future hole of the umbilicus on the median line and to use the length of the umbilicus to reach the right place.

The cutaneous flap is closed under tension after raising the patient to the sitting position. Double drainage is recommended. At the end of the closure, the color of the flap should be checked to verify the quality of blood supply. If there is any doubt, it is necessary to sit the patient up a little more and remove the dubious area.

7.9.2 Free Flaps

a. TRAM Free Flaps

TRAM free flaps require the use of microsurgical procedures. These flaps reduce the amount of muscle tissue removed. There are three different types of free flaps:

1. In the classic free flap, a small portion of muscle together with the skin paddle is removed at the level of the perforator vessels. The inferior epigastric vessels are skeletonized and prepared for microvascular anastomosis.
2. In the perforator flap, the perforators up to the skin paddle are skeletonized, without any muscle removal.
3. The third type of abdominal free flap is based on the external iliac vessels, which are available anatomically in only about 70% of cases.

b. Superior and inferior gluteus maximus muscle cutaneous flaps.

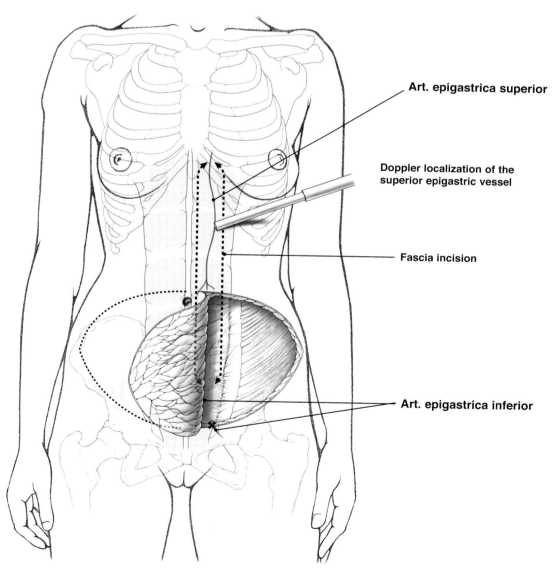

Art. epigastrica superior

Doppler localization of the superior epigastric vessel

Fascia incision

Art. epigastrica inferior

Fig. 7.16. Pedicle TRAM flap reconstruction

Fig. 7.17. Complete harvesting
of one pedicle

7

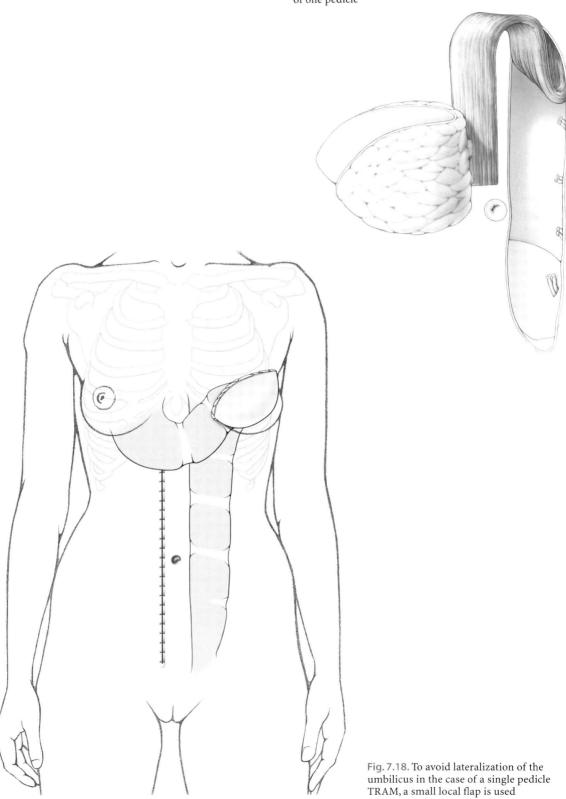

Fig. 7.18. To avoid lateralization of the
umbilicus in the case of a single pedicle
TRAM, a small local flap is used

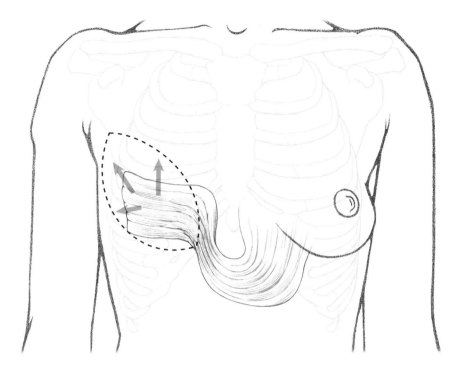

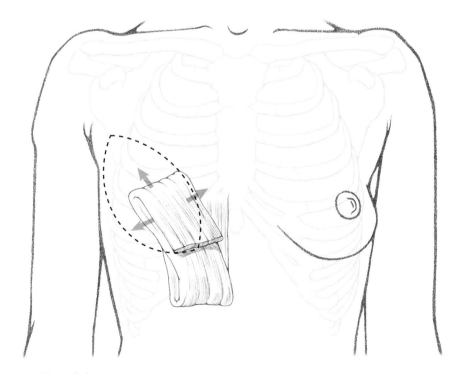

Fig. 7.19. Rotation of the pedicle

7

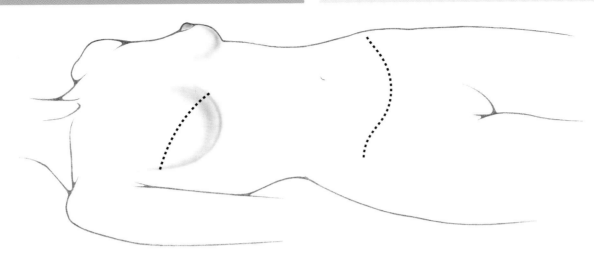

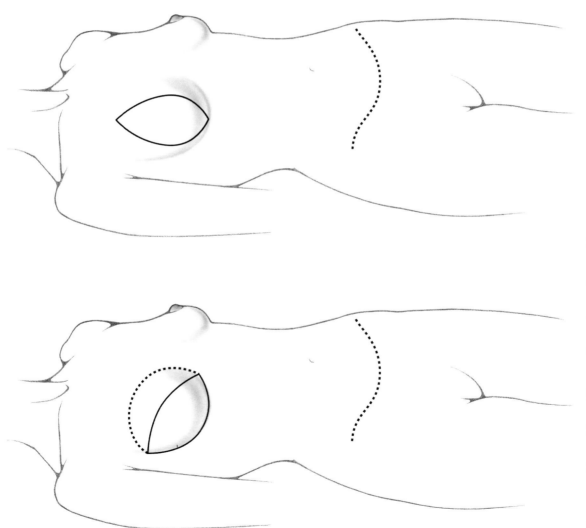

Fig. 7.20. Positions of the paddle according to the previous positions

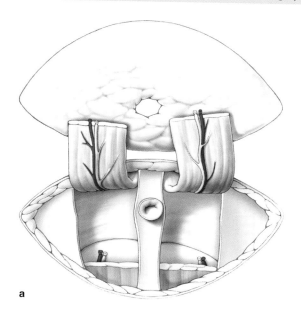

a

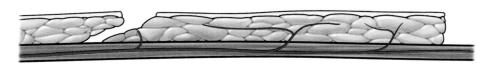

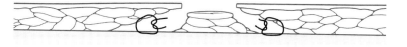

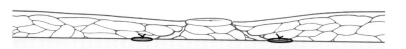

b

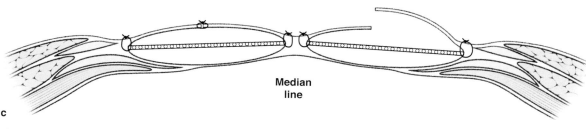

Median line

c

Fig. 7.21a–c. a Bipedicle flap. b Umbilical closure. c Abdominal closure

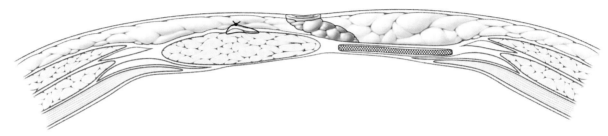

Fig. 7.22. Abdominal closure TRAM. Centralization of the umbilicus in the case of a single pedicle TRAM

7

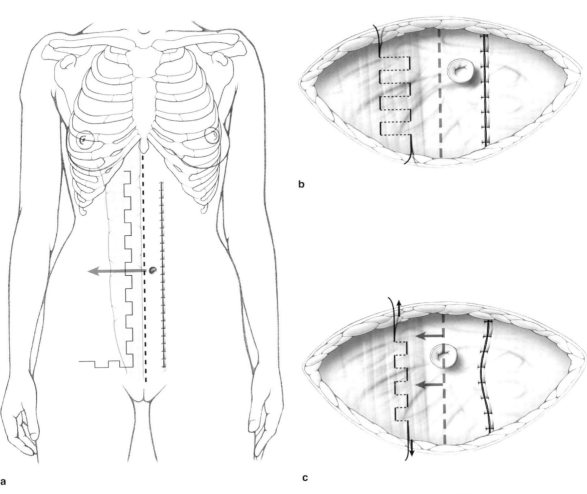

a   c

Fig. 7.23a–c. Left pedicle TRAM with suture on the right rectus sheath in order to centralize the umbilicus

7.10 Nipple Reconstruction

The creation of a nipple–areola complex following breast reconstruction improves the cosmetic outcome, and many patients may request such a procedure. The most popular technique for nipple reconstruction combines a tattoo procedure with a small triangular skin flap that is often referred to as a skate flap, illustrated in Fig. 7.24. The location of the areolar should be drawn preoperatively with the patient in the standing position to check for bilateral symmetry of the nipple–areola complex. The nipple–areola reconstruction is generally performed as a second-stage procedure under local anesthesia. The tattooing should be done prior to reconstructing the nipple. A skin flap is then developed and folded on itself and sutured with 4–0 absorbable sutures, as shown in the accompanying illustrations. The angle of the skin flap should be oriented appropriately if it is in the vicinity of the previous mastectomy scar (Fig. 7.25).

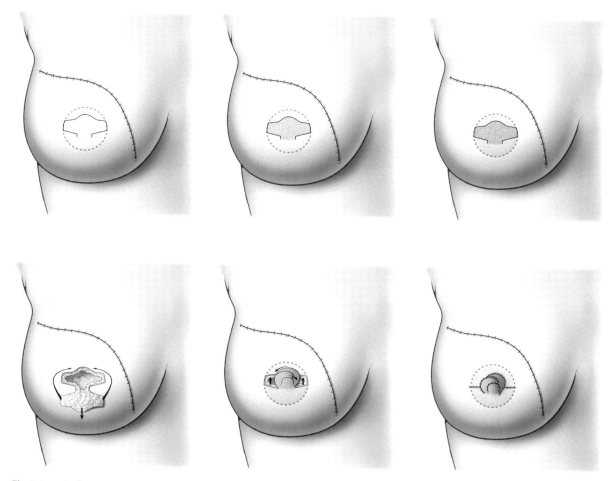

Fig. 7.24. Nipple–areola reconstruction (color of the areola and the nipple is obtained by tattooing the surface of the circle)

7

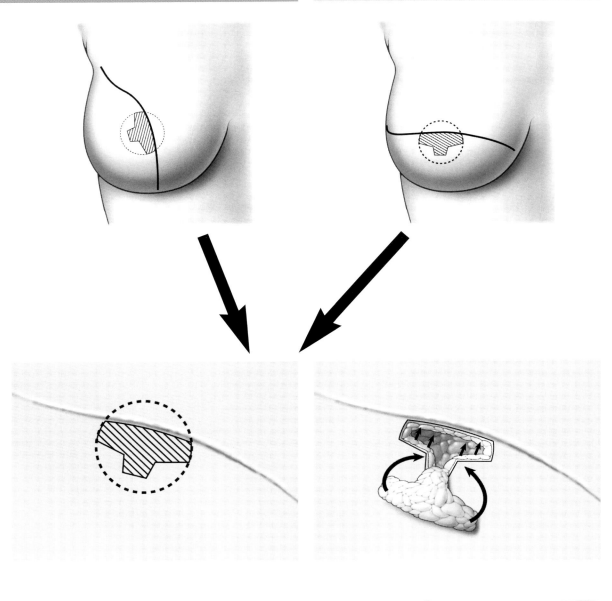

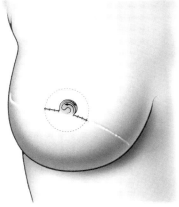

Fig. 7.25. Nipple–areola reconstruction in the vicinity of the previous mastectomy scar

7.11 Thoracoepigastric Cutaneous Flap for Large Thoracic Wall Defects

Local recurrences following mastectomy for breast cancer will generally require extensive skin and muscle resection. The latissimus dorsi or TRAM flaps are often used to close such defects. However, when the defect is not too large, a thoracoepigastric cutaneous flap can be used. The blood supply for this flap is derived from the epigastric perforators and, as shown in the accompanying illustrations (Fig. 7.26), the flap can be developed horizontally, with its superior end towards the axilla. The fascia of the abdominal muscles should remain attached to the flap to preserve its blood supply. After rotation of the flap, the chest wall defect should be closed with the patient placed in a semi-sitting position on the operating room table to facilitate advancement of the flap.

Also, chest wall defects can be closed with mesh, using the suspension technique described in Figs. 7.9a, b and 7.10a, b.

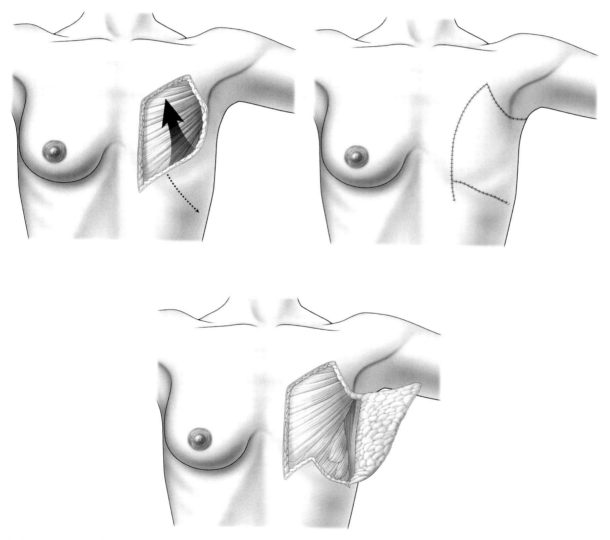

Fig. 7.26. Thoraco-axillary cutaneous flap for large thoracic defects

7.12 Partial (or Total) Reconstruction with Omental Flaps

Local recurrences following mastectomy for breast cancer can also be managed with omental flaps (Fig. 7.27). Following resection of the area of local recurrence, an omental flap can be used to cover the defect. The omentum is one of the most vascularized tissues of the body and provides excellent material to close huge defects, particularly after radiotherapy.

The omentum should be mobilized with a pedicle consisting of the right gastroepiploic artery and vein. It should be detached from the greater curvature of the stomach. This dissection can also be done by endoscopy, with the omental flap pulled up to the surface of the thoracic wall through a small peritoneal hole in the epigastric area. It can also be used as a free flap because the vessels are wide and can therefore be easily anastomosed. In selected cases, the omental flap can also be used for partial breast reconstruction.

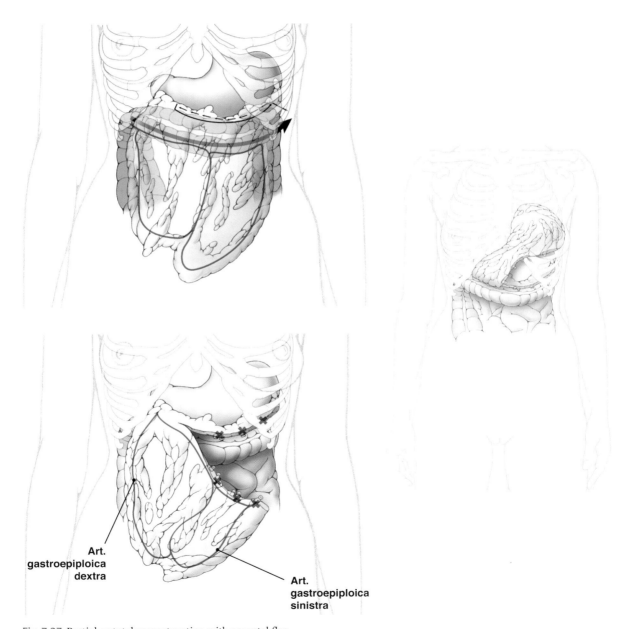

Art. gastroepiploica dextra

Art. gastroepiploica sinistra

Fig. 7.27. Partial or total reconstruction with omental flap

7.13 Reduction Mammoplasty

Heavy, pendulous breasts are often a source of chronic pain and discomfort for many women. Although women may request reduction mammoplasty to relieve pain and discomfort, many also hope that the procedure will improve their appearance.

Prior to undertaking breast reduction mammoplasty, the surgeon should document several measurements that are useful in the procedure. These measurements are indicated in Fig. 7.28.

Additionally, the breasts should be appropriately marked with the patient in the standing position, indicating the planned incision pattern, as depicted in the accompanying illustration (Fig. 7.29).

As shown in the accompanying illustrations, reduction mammoplasty can be performed using a vertical technique, where a superior pedicle is left intact, providing blood supply to the nipple–areola complex (Fig. 7.30a). Alternatively, the procedure can be performed with an inferior pedicle providing the necessary blood supply to the nipple–areola complex (Fig. 7.30b).

The drawings on this page illustrate both the superior pedicle technique and the inferior pedicle technique. Specifically, these drawings depict the contour of the breast tissue specimen that is obtained after using the superior pedicle technique and the contour of the breast tissue specimen that is obtained after using the inferior pedicle technique for reduction mammoplasty (Fig. 7.30c, d).

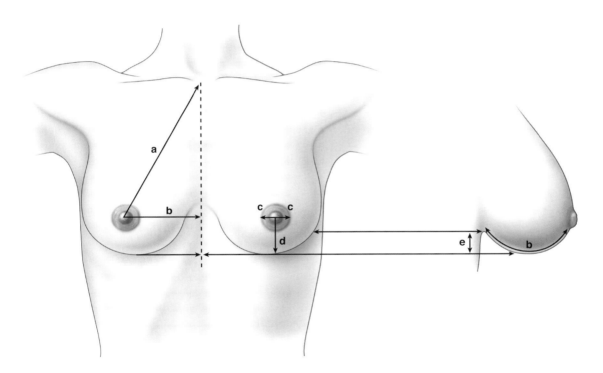

Fig. 7.28. Measurements required prior to reduction mammoplasty. a=19–21 cm; b=9–11 cm; c=4–5 cm; d=5–8 cm; e=0–2 cm

7

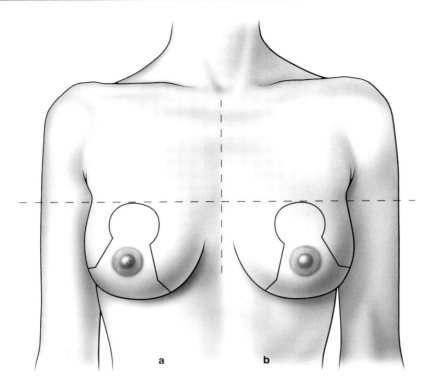

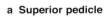
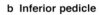

a Superior pedicle

b Inferior pedicle

Fig. 7.29. Reduction mammoplasty

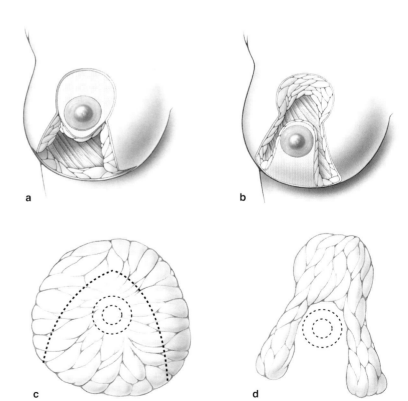

Fig. 7.30a–d. Reduction mammoplasty

7.14 Reduction Mammoplasty: Vertical Technique (Lejour)

Figure 7.31 depicts a surgeon's preoperative drawing for a reduction mammoplasty, utilizing the vertical scar technique (Lejour). The drawing shows the limit of the supra-areolar de-epithelialization (1, in Fig. 7.32a), the medial limit of infra-areolar de-epithelialization (2, in Fig. 7.31a), the lateral limit of infra-areolar de-epithelialization (3, in Fig. 7.31b), and the inferior aspect of the resection (4, in Fig. 7.31c).

The accompanying illustrations briefly summarize the key features of the reduction mammoplasty utilizing the vertical technique (Lejour). A margin of tissue around the nipple–areola complex is de-epithelialized (1, in Fig. 7.31a). The surgeon undermines a wide area of tissue anterior to the serratus anterior and pectoralis major muscles. Breast tissue in the inferior quadrant is then resected (Fig. 7.32). Glandular tissue is then re-approximated with absorbable stitches (Fig. 7.33). The skin edges are re-approximated with interrupted 3–0 Monocryl stitches (Fig. 7.33). These stitches are also used to re-approximate the

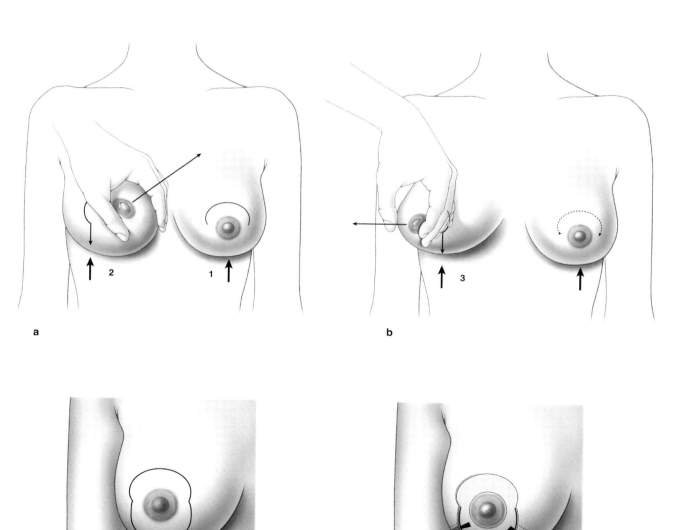

Fig. 7.31a–d. Reduction mammoplasty; vertical scar technique (Lejour)

de-epithelialized tissue around the nipple–areola complex and to close the inferior vertical incision.

The accompanying illustrations further depict key aspects of the reduction mammoplasty using the vertical technique (Lejour). Seen here is the appearance of the breast after de-epithelialization with a section of the glandular tissue shown inferiorly. The illustration above (Fig. 7.30a, b) depicts the appearance of the breast tissue after glandular resection. The illustration below (Fig. 7.30c, d) depicts the appearance of the glandular tissue that has been resected and sent to the pathologist.

This illustration (Fig. 7.30a–d) further demonstrates the technique of wide retroglandular undermining anterior to the pectoralis major muscle. This undermining allows the surgeon to eventually restore the continuity of the gland after resection, and also to bimanually palpate the breast to check for the presence of any tumors.

Seen in this illustration (Fig. 7.30a–d) is the appearance of the breast after peri-areolar and inferior de-epithelialization, with undermining of the lower glandular tissue.

7

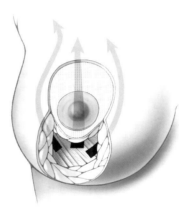

Fig. 7.32. Reduction mammoplasty; vertical scar technique (Lejour)

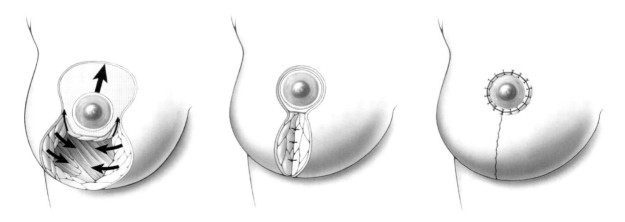

Fig. 7.33. Reduction mammoplasty; vertical scar technique (Lejour)

7.15 Reduction Mammoplasty: Inferior Pedicle Technique

If the inferior pedicle technique of reduction mammoplasty is utilized, then the blood supply to the nipple–areola complex is derived from a pyramid of tissue along the inferior aspect of the breast.

The accompanying illustrations provide an overview of the technique. An inferior pedicle is de-epithelialized from the nipple–areola complex down to the inframammary fold (Fig. 7.34a). The surgeon then sharply divides tissue along the medial and lateral borders of this inferior pedicle, and resects tissue medial and lateral to the pedicle (away from the pedicle), as shown in Fig. 7.34b, c. The glandular tissue is then re-approximated with absorbable sutures, and the medical and lateral flaps are advanced and closed along the inframammary fold (Fig. 7.34d).

The appearance of the resected breast specimen is also shown in the accompanying illustration (Fig. 7.34c).

Reduction mammoplasty utilizing the inferior pedicle technique is further illustrated in Fig. 7.35a–c, utilizing the Thorek technique. These illustrations depict the appearance of the vertical and horizontal scars utilized for the operation, and again show the appearance of the accompanying breast specimen that is obtained following the resection (Fig. 7.35b). Also seen is the technique of amputation of the nipple–areola complex and grafting of the complex onto the glandular tissue after complete skin suture (Fig. 7.35c) (Thorek).

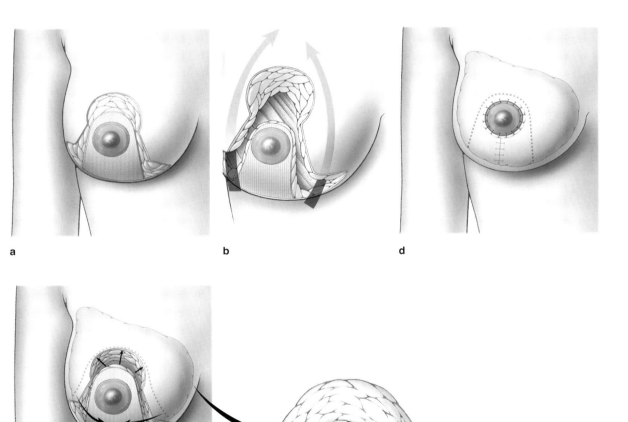

a   b   d

c

Fig. 7.34a–d. Reduction mammoplasty; inferior pedicle technique

7

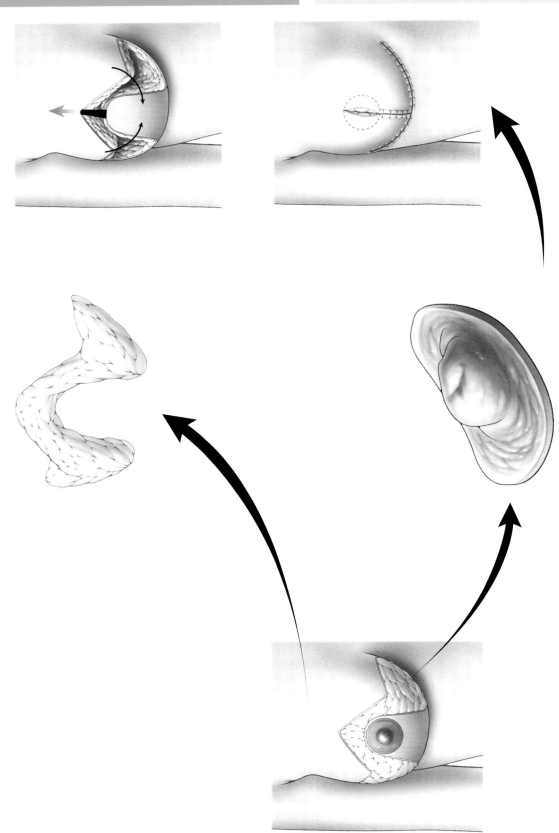

Fig. 7.35a–c. Reduction mammoplasty; inferior pedicle technique with vertical and horizontal scar (Thorek)

7.16 Round Block Technique of Reduction Mammoplasty

Figure 7.36 depicts the round block technique for reduction mammoplasty. As shown, a rim of tissue around the nipple–areola complex is de-epithelialized, and tissue from the inferior quadrant of the breast is resected. The defect in the inferior quadrant of the breast is then re-approximated with absorbable interrupted sutures.

The de-epithelialized skin around the nipple–areola complex is re-approximated with a running 2–0 Monocryl or a nonabsorbable subcuticular stitch. A second purse string suture is done with 4/0 Monocryl to close the skin.

The appearance of the resected breast tissue is also depicted (Fig. 7.36).

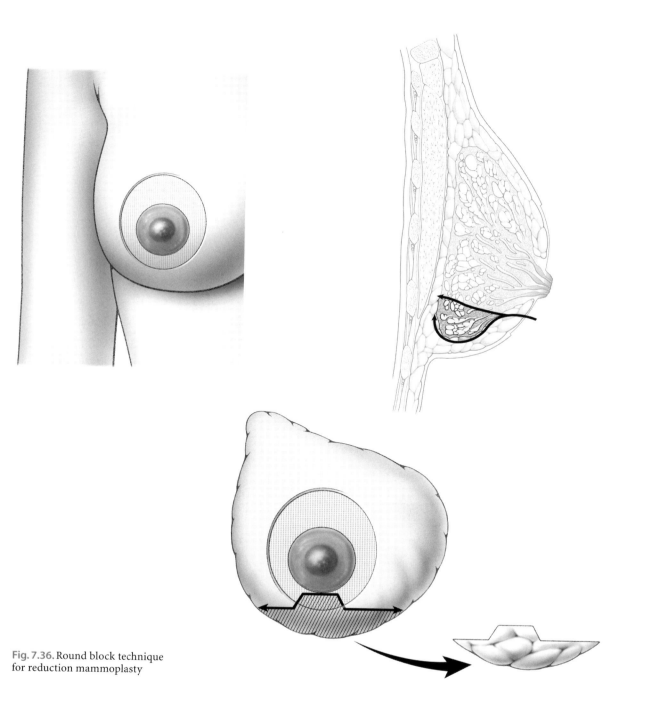

Fig. 7.36. Round block technique for reduction mammoplasty

7

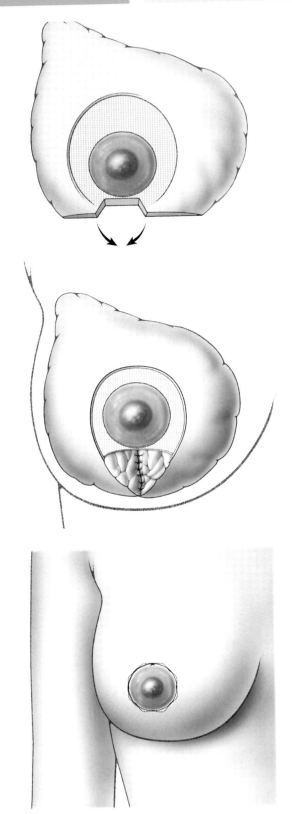

Fig. 7.36. Continued

7.17 Breast Ptosis Classification

Breast ptosis is defined by the position of the nipple–areola complex relative to the inframammary crease. This classification scheme, developed by Regnault, is illustrated in the accompanying diagrams.

In the normal breast, the entire breast, including the nipple–areola complex, lies above the level of the inframammary crease (Fig. 7.37a).

In a patient with minor ptosis, the nipple lies at the level of the inframammary crease (Fig. 7.37b).

If the nipple lies below the level of the inframammary crease but remains above the lower contour of the breast gland, then this is referred to as moderate ptosis (Fig. 7.37c).

In a patient with severe ptosis, the nipple lies below the inframammary crease and along the lower contour of the breast (Fig. 7.37d).

In pseudoptosis, the nipple is above the level of the inframammary crease, but loose skin droops below the level of the crease (Fig. 7.37e).

Parenchymal maldistribution refers to a situation where the nipple and the lower aspect of the breast droop below the inframammary crease, as shown in the accompanying diagram (Fig. 7.37f).

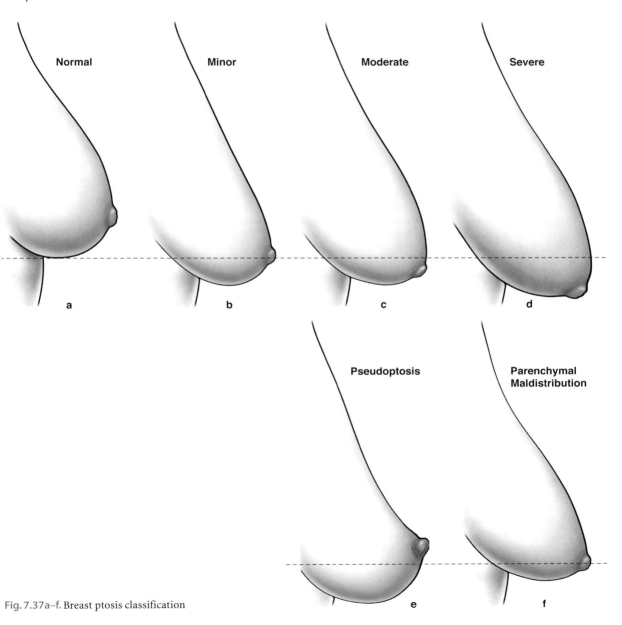

Fig. 7.37a–f. Breast ptosis classification

7.18 Mastopexy

A mastopexy, also referred to as a "breast lift," is indicated to correct the more severe forms of ptosis, and this procedure is described later in this text. If a patient presents with minor ptosis or pseudoptosis, an area cephalad to the nipple–areola complex is de-epithelialized, and the nipple–areola complex is then advanced.

Patients who will benefit most from mastopexy are generally those with moderate or severe ptosis. There are several techniques available that can correct this ptosis, and these are illustrated in the accompanying pages.

Mastopexy is sometimes performed with deep fixation of the breast tissue to the underlying pectoralis major muscle. In this technique, a plane is dissected inferiorly between the breast and skin. Also, a plane between the breast and the skin is dissected superiorly, and this is extended posteriorly for a short distance to create a plane between the breast and pectoralis major muscle. Along the superior aspect, a few stitches are then placed to fix the breast to the underlying pectoralis major muscle. This serves to lift the breast up, improving its projection.

This technique often produces an immediate good result, but the mastopexy is generally not stable, and long-term results are often not good.

In the following pages, more suitable techniques for mastopexy are described and illustrated.

7.19 Round Block Technique for Mastopexy

Figures 7.38 and 7.39 depict the round block technique for mastopexy. The patient who presents with a significant degree of ptosis undergoes periareolar de-epithelialization (Fig. 7.38a). Following this, there are two options available. A single purse string suture can be placed, bringing the edges of the de-epithelialized surface together (Fig. 7.38b, c). The surface of the breast adjacent to the nipple–areola complex will now appear flattened, giving the appearance of a "tomato shape breast" (Fig. 7.38d). This technique is useful for making very small corrections.

Alternatively, following de-epithelialization around the nipple–areola complex, the surgeon may elect to model the glandular tissue in the lower quadrant underneath the de-epithelialized area (Fig. 7.38e, f). The gland is transected in order to obtain two glandular flaps which will cross each other and be fixed to the pectoral fascia in order to reduce the diameter of the base of the gland and increase the projection of the breast (Fig. 7.38g). The skin edges of the de-epithelialized area are approximated. This generally results in a good final projection of the breast, as seen in this illustration (Fig. 7.38h).

Figure 7.39 demonstrates the use of dermal flaps (de-epithelialized skin) to fix the breast to the pectoralis major muscle (somewhat like an internal bra). This results in an improved projection of the breast. As illustrated, the dermis is undermined, creating a dermal flap, which is brought down to the pectoralis major muscle. There, the dermal flap is sutured to the muscle (Fig. 7.39a, b).

Alternatively, if the dermal flap is too short, a semi-absorbable mesh is used (Goes). One end of the Vicryl mesh is sutured anteriorly to the dermal flap, and the other end is sutured posteriorly to the pectoralis major muscle (Fig. 7.39c, d). The skin edges are approximated with a 3–0 Monocryl subcuticular stitch. The final suture lines are depicted in the accompanying illustration (Fig. 7.39c, d).

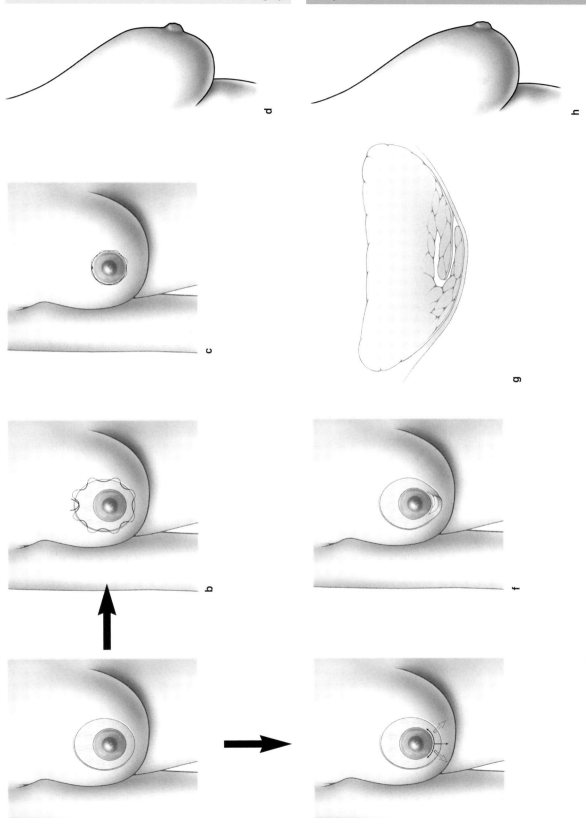

Fig. 7.38a–h. Round block technique for mastopexy

7

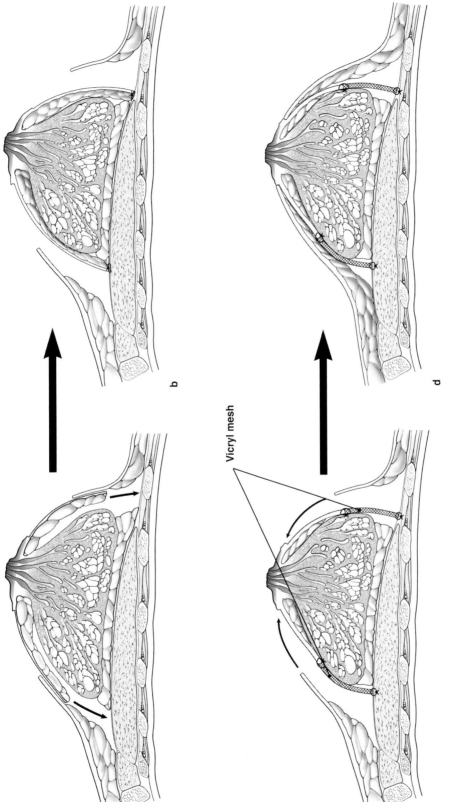

Vicryl mesh

Fig. 7.39. Round block technique for mastopexy

7.20 Mastopexy: Oblique Technique (DuFourmentel)

In this technique (Fig. 7.40), a rim of tissue around the nipple–areola complex is de-epithelialized. After de-epithelialization, a section of breast tissue is re-sected inferiorly, and the adjacent breast tissue is undermined. The defect in the breast is then closed with absorbable sutures, and the skin edges are approximated with a 3–0 Monocryl subcuticular stitch. Also, the de-epithelialized area around the nipple–areola complex is approximated with a running absorbable stitch.

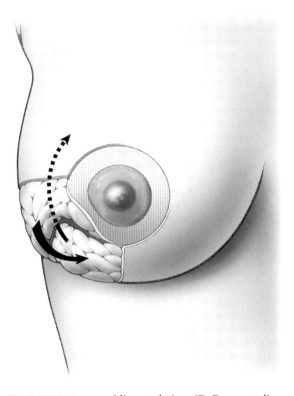
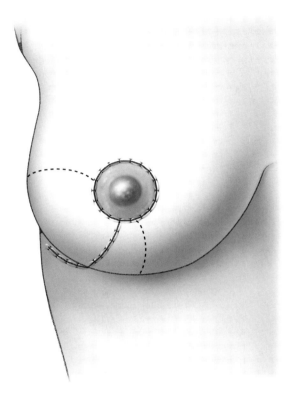

Fig. 7.40. Mastopexy; oblique technique (DuFourmentel)

7.21 Augmentation Mammoplasty

Augmentation mammoplasty is one of the most common cosmetic procedures performed by plastic surgeons. The procedure is particularly popular among younger women, and the illustrations on these pages provide only a brief overview of the various procedures.

As shown in the accompanying illustrations, there are three surgical approaches available for augmentation mammoplasty. These are the axillary, periareolar, and inframammary fold approaches (Fig. 7.41a–c). As shown, all three approaches allow the surgeon to create a plane between the breast and the anterior aspect of the pectoralis major muscle, or, alternatively, between the posterior aspect of the muscle and the chest wall.

Figure 7.42 shows that the prostheses for augmentation mammoplasty can be placed as either submammary or subpectoral implants.

As depicted in Fig. 7.43, patients with breast asymmetry may elect to undergo augmentation mammoplasty. In this instance, the prosthesis is generally placed in the submammary position (anterior to the pectoralis major muscle).

7

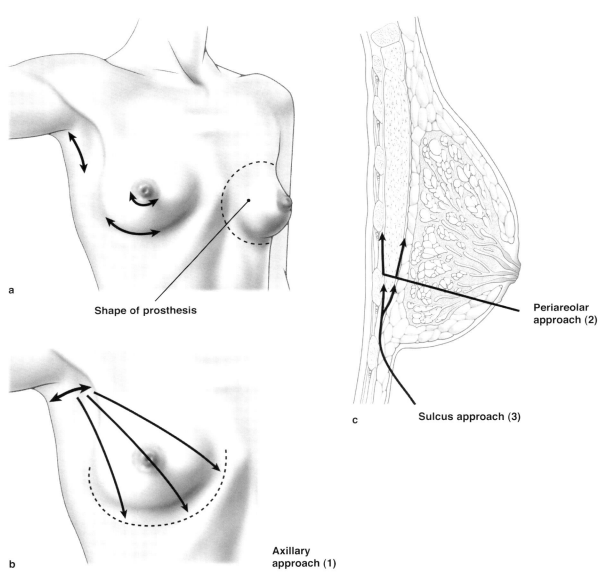

a

Shape of prosthesis

b

Axillary approach (1)

c

Periareolar approach (2)

Sulcus approach (3)

Fig. 7.41a–c. Surgical approaches for augmentation mammoplasty

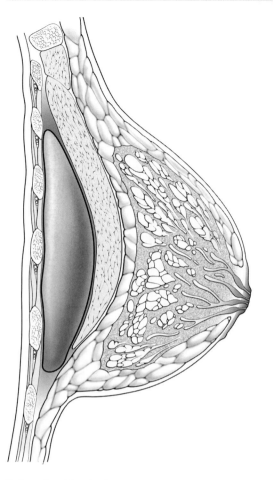
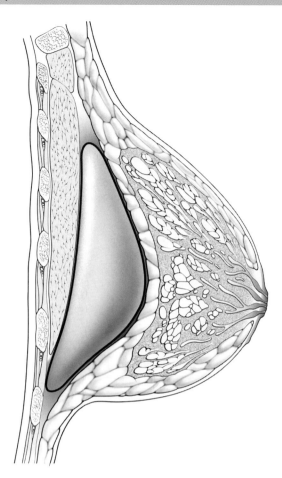

Subpectoral implant   **Prepectoral implant**

Fig. 7.42. Augmentation mammoplasty

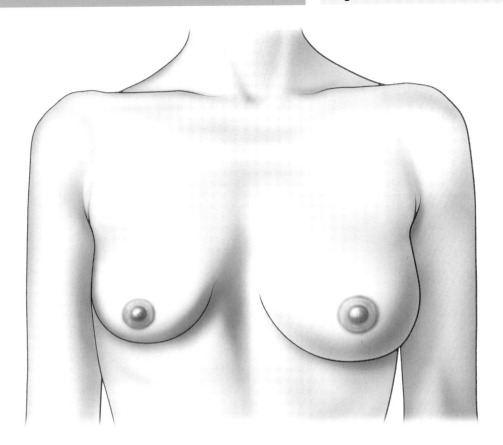

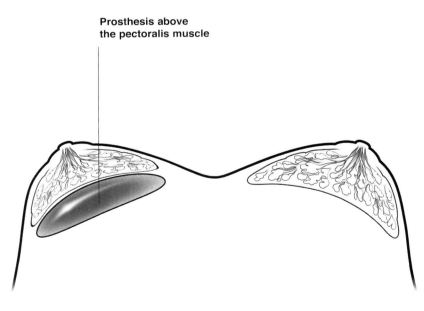

**Prosthesis above
the pectoralis muscle**

Fig. 7.43. Augmentation mammoplasty for breast asymmetry

7.22 Nipple Plasty for Inverted Nipple

The technique of nipple plasty for inverted nipple is described in the accompanying illustrations. The procedure begins with a curvilinear incision adjacent to the inverted nipple (Fig. 7.44b). The dissection is then continued posteriorly as shown, so that the inverted nipple can be lifted up with a skin hook (Fig. 7.44c). An absorbable stitch is then placed around the nipple after it has been lifted up (Fig. 7.44d), and this is securely tied down.

A plastic syringe that has been cut is then placed over the nipple. As depicted in the illustration, two 3–0 Prolene stitches are then passed (one on each side of the cut syringe). These extend from the nipple, through the plastic syringe, and are then tied down on the skin (Fig. 7.44e). In this way, the nipple that has been brought up is secured, and is kept in this position for about 10 days, until the wounds heal.

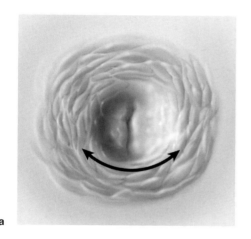

a

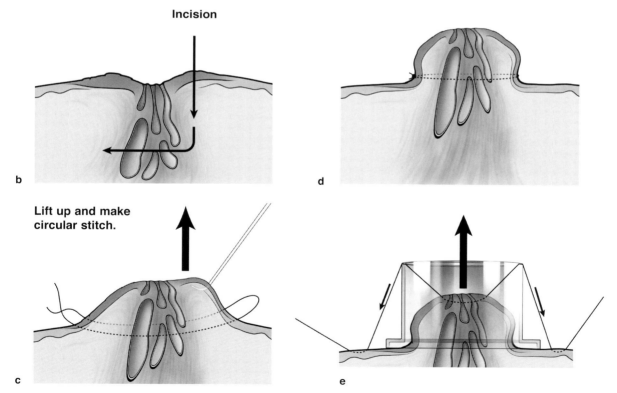

Incision

b

Lift up and make circular stitch.

c

d

e

Fig. 7.44. Nipple plasty for inverted nipple

References

1. Delay E, Gounot N, Bouillot A, Zlatoff P, Rivoire M (1998) Autologous latissimus breast reconstruction: a 3-year clinical experience with 100 patients. Plast Reconstr Surg 102(5):1461–1478
2. Coleman DJ, Sharpe DT, Naylor IL, Chander CL, Cross SE (1993) The role of the contractile fibroblast in the capsules around tissue expanders and implants. Br J Plastic Surg 46:547–556
3. Rietjens M, Garusi C, Lanfrey E, Petit JY (1997) Cutaneous suspension: immediate breast reconstruction with abdominal cutaneous advancement using a non-resorptive mesh. Preliminary results and report of 28 cases. [French] Ann Chir Plast Esthet 42(2):177–182

7

Subject Index

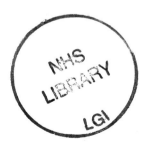

Printing and Binding: Stürtz GmbH, Würzburg